Rare Diseases - Diagnostic and Therapeutic Odyssey

Edited by Mani T. Valarmathi

Published in London, United Kingdom

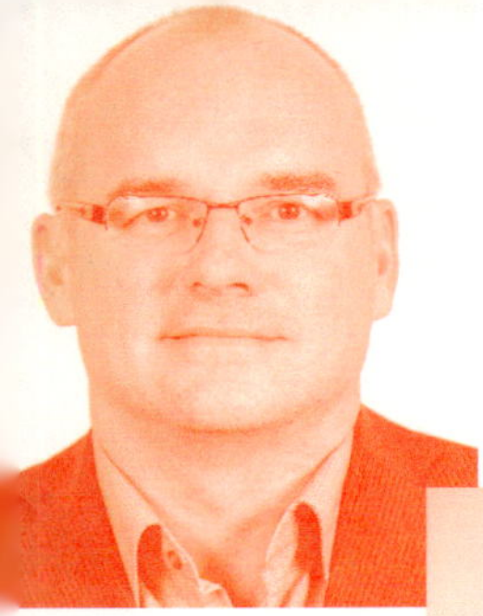
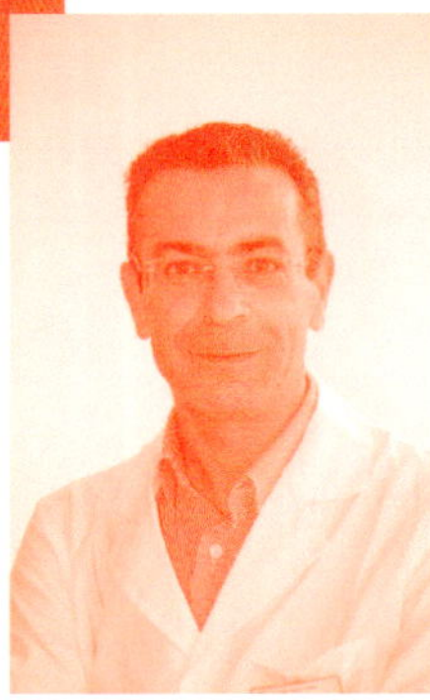
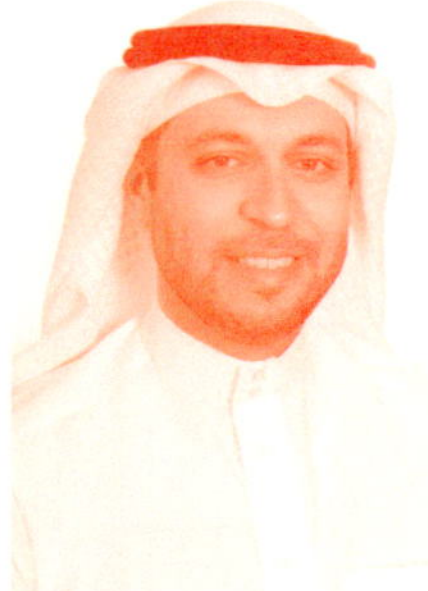
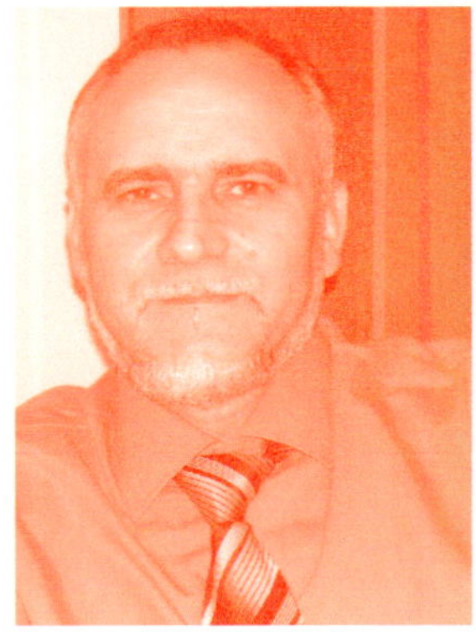
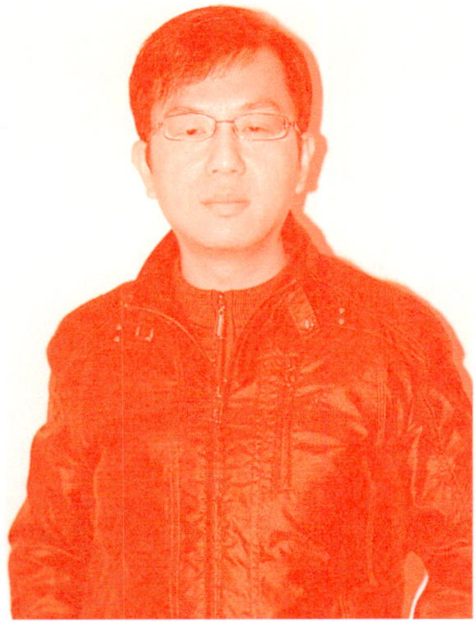
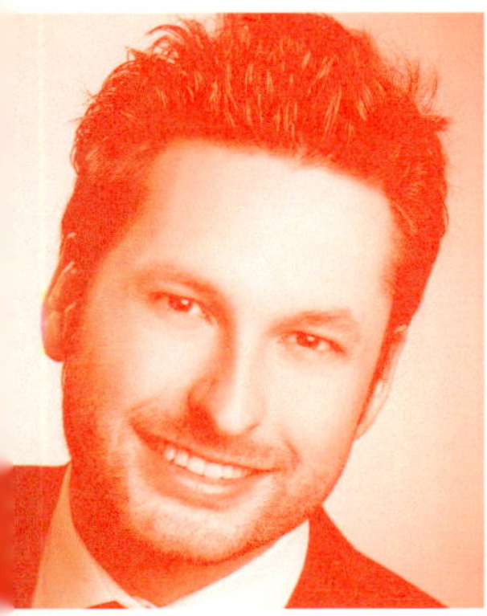
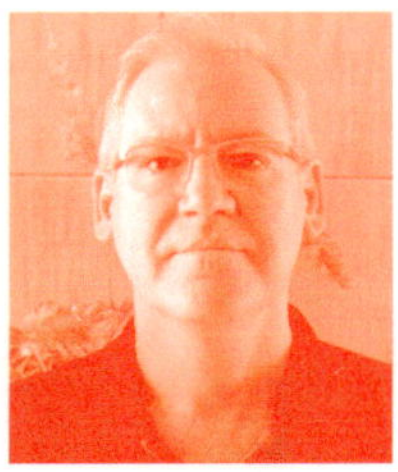

IntechOpen

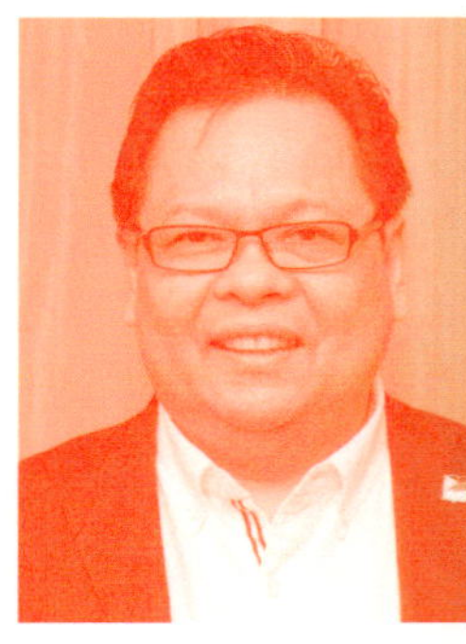
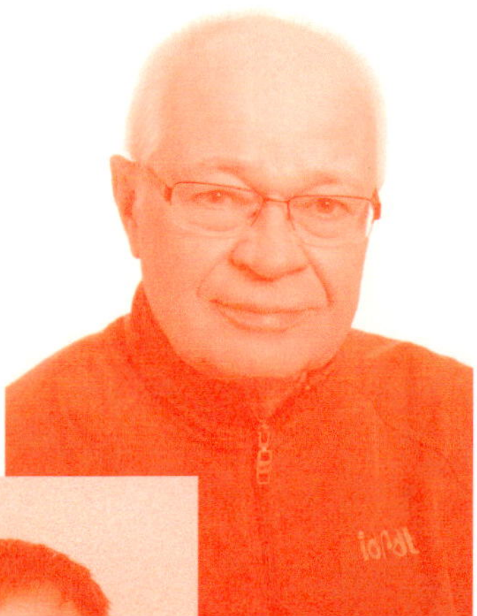
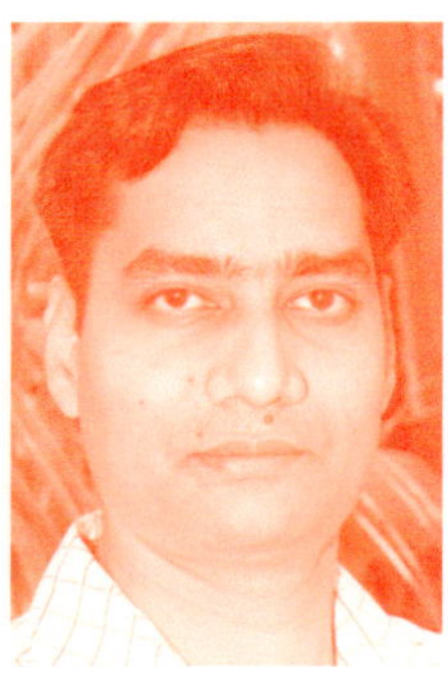
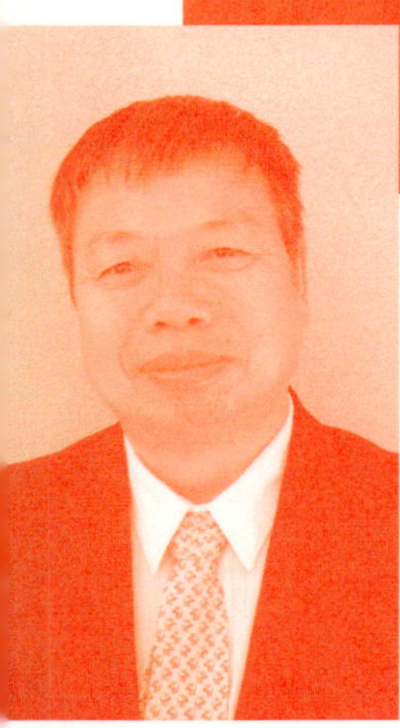
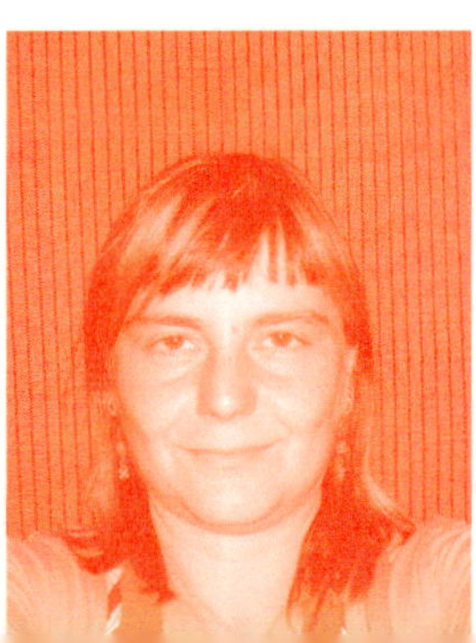
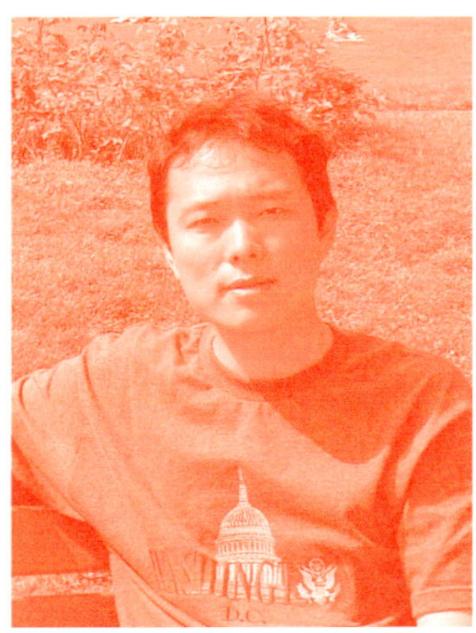

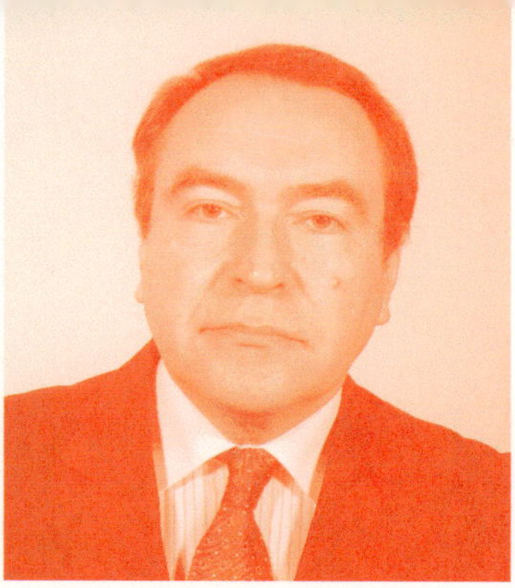
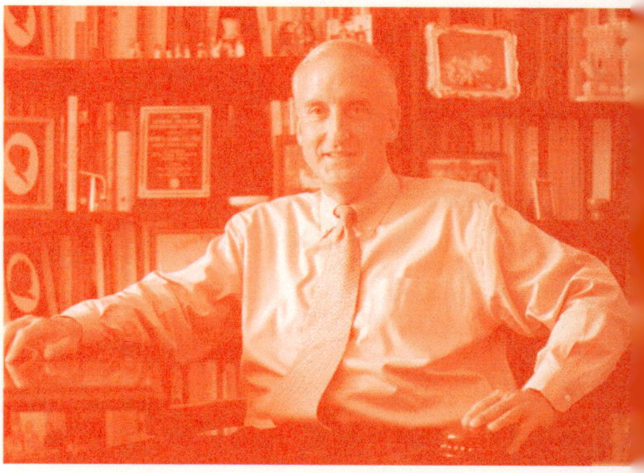
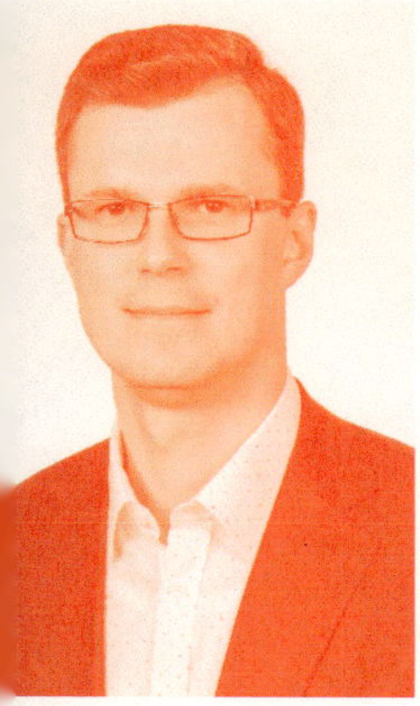
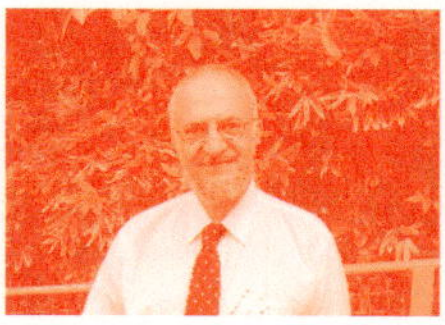
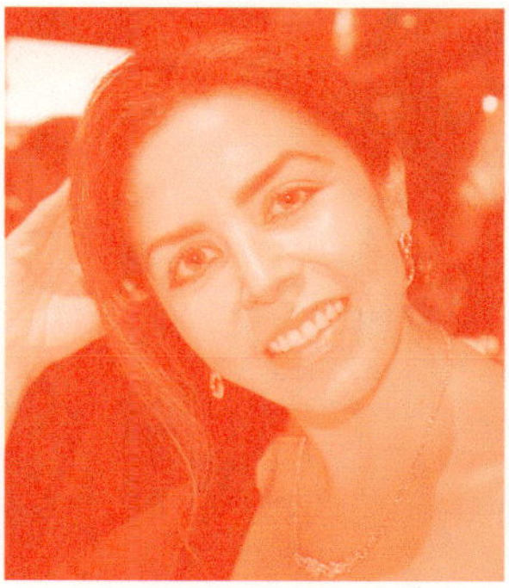

Supporting open minds since 2005

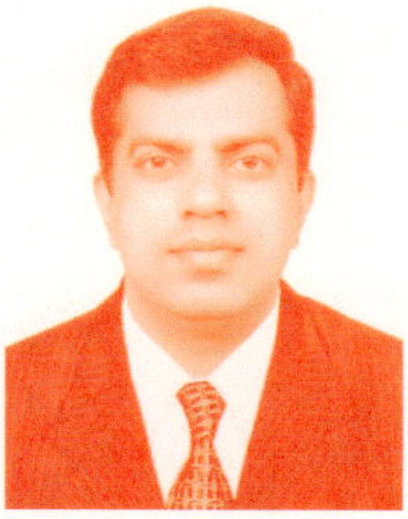
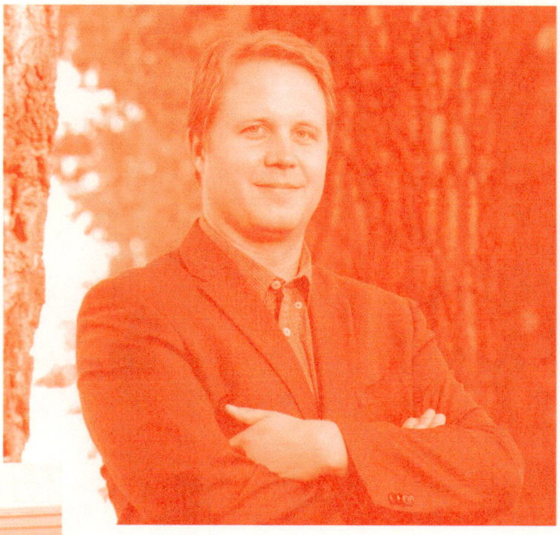
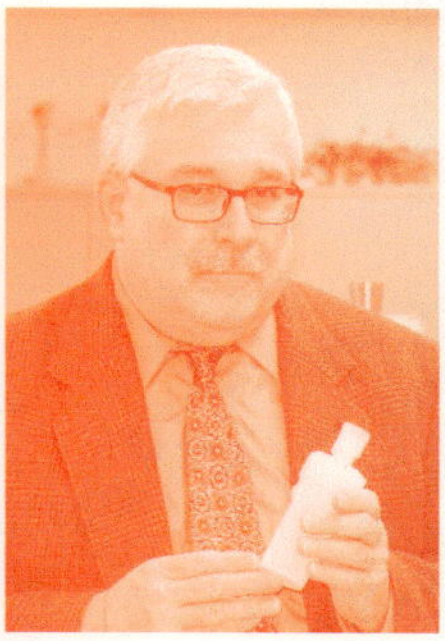
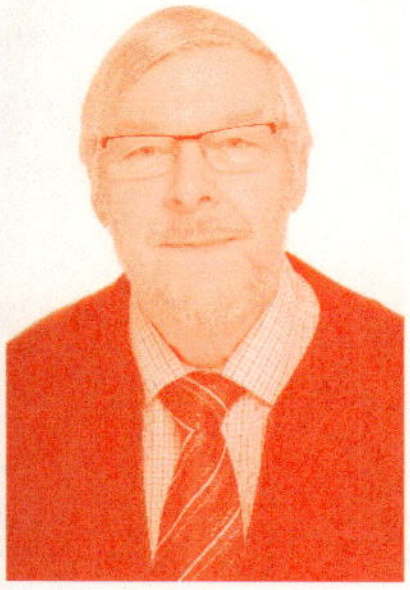
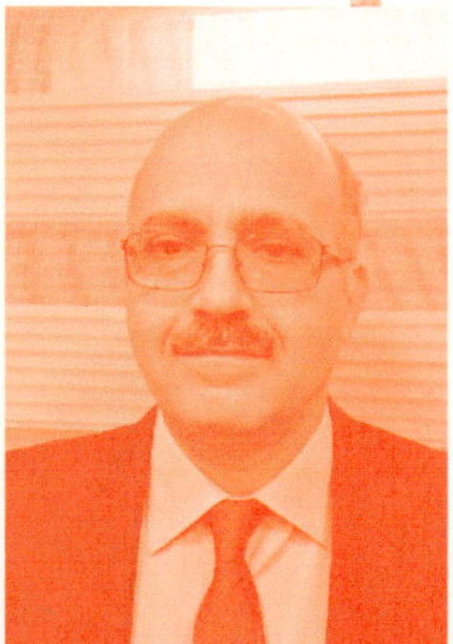
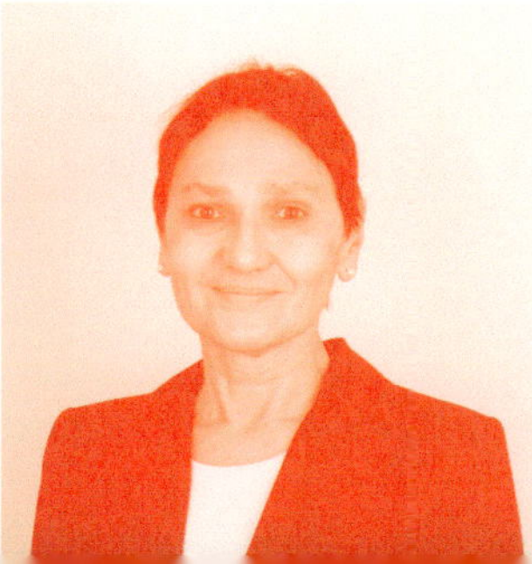
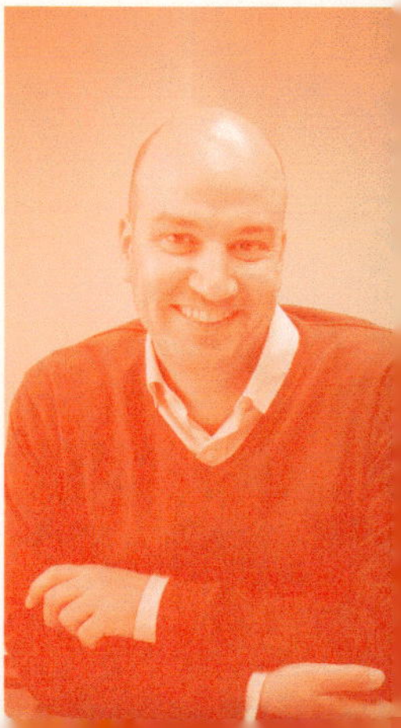

Rare Diseases - Diagnostic and Therapeutic Odyssey
http://dx.doi.org/10.5772/intechopen.92919
Edited by Mani T. Valarmathi

Contributors
Milen Minkov, Katharina Sterlich, Vadim Gorodetskiy, Massimiliano Mazza, Fabio Nicolini, Verena Wally, Ulrich Koller, Christina Gruber, Josefina Piñón Hofbauer, Iris Gratz, Piotr Fiedor, Magdalena Nita, Shiyu Wang, Shaleindra Singh, Mani T. Valarmathi, Jacek Pliszczyński, Andrzej Eljaszewicz, Marcin Moniuszko, Tomasz Ołdak, Katarzyna Woźniak, Sławomir Majewski, Cezary Kowalewski, Artur Kamiński, Dariusz Śladowski, Zbigniew Zimek, Maciej Kosieradzki

First published in London, United Kingdom, 2021 by IntechOpen
IntechOpen is the global imprint of INTECHOPEN LIMITED, registered in England and Wales, registration number: 11086078, 5 Princes Gate Court, London, SW7 2QJ, United Kingdom
Printed in Croatia

British Library Cataloguing-in-Publication Data
A catalogue record for this book is available from the British Library

Additional hard and PDF copies can be obtained from orders@intechopen.com

Rare Diseases - Diagnostic and Therapeutic Odyssey
Edited by Mani T. Valarmathi
p. cm.
Print ISBN 978-1-83962-930-3
Online ISBN 978-1-83969-412-7
eBook (PDF) ISBN 978-1-83969-413-4

For EU product safety concerns:
IN TECH d.o.o., Prolaz Marije Krucifikse Kozulić 3, 51000 Rijeka, Croatia, info@intechopen.com or visit our website at intechopen.com.

Meet the editor

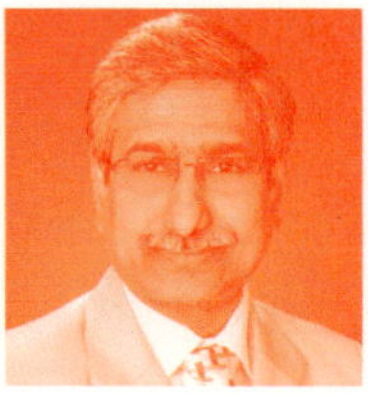

Mani T. Valarmathi is currently Director of Research and Development at Religen Inc., a Life Science Company in Pennsylvania, USA. He began his scientific career as a cancer geneticist, but soon became captivated with the emerging and translational fields of stem cell biology, tissue engineering, and regenerative medicine. After obtaining a bachelor's degree in Chemistry from the University of Madras, Chennai, Tamil Nadu, India, he obtained an MBBS in Medicine and Surgery and MD in Pathology from the same university, as well as a Ph.D. in Medical Biotechnology from All-India Institute of Medical Sciences, New Delhi, India. Over the past two decades, he has had extensive experience in research on various types of stem cells, and his research work has been focused on creating bioengineered human 3D vascularized tissues constructs for implantation purposes. At present, much of his research is directed towards developing innovative molecular genetic testing for precision and genetic medicine. He is a member of many prestigious national and international professional societies and scientific organizations, including the International Society for Stem Cell Research (ISSCR), Tissue Engineering and Regenerative Medicine International Society (TERMIS), American Association for Cancer Research (AACR), American Society for Investigative Pathology (ASIP), American Society for Clinical Pathology (ASCP), American Chemical Society (ACS), European Society of Cardiology (ESC), International Society for Heart Research (ISHR), American Society of Gene & Cell Therapy (ASGCT), and American Heart Association (AHA).

Contents

Preface

A rare disease is any disease or condition that affects a small percentage of the population. In the United States alone, more than 7000 rare diseases affect more than thirty million people. Many rare conditions are not only life-threatening or chronically debilitating diseases, but most do not have appropriate treatments, rendering them incurable. As a result, drug, biological, and device development in the case of rare diseases is challenging for many reasons, including the complex biology and the lack of critical understanding of the natural course of many rare diseases. In addition, the inherently fewer population of patients with a rare disease can also make conducting clinical trials difficult.

In recent years, there has been substantial development in the area of rare disease research and its clinical applications, for instance, rare disease biology and genomics; epidemiology and preventions; early detection and screening; and diagnosis and treatment. In addition, the advent of various emerging technologies, such as genome editing technology, stem cell technology, and tissue engineering and regenerative medicine, as well the integrated knowledge gained from such studies, enhances our understanding of rare diseases and produces novel insights that could lead to the development and timely deployment of novel clinical and/or therapeutic interventions.

In this context, this book consolidates the recent advances in rare disease biology and therapeutics covering a wide spectrum of interrelated topics in a timely fashion. It disseminates this essential knowledge in a comprehensible way to a greater scientific and clinical audience as well as patients, caregivers, and drug and device manufacturers, especially to support rare disease product development.

Written by leading experts in basic science and clinical care, this book consists of seven chapters over four sections. The first section introduces rare diseases, emphasizing the current challenges and future perspectives within the context of the advancement of genetic and precision medicine. The second section deals with selected rare disease syndromes, such as Felty's syndrome, a rare immune system disease, and Löfgren's syndrome, a rare acute form of sarcoidosis.

The third section discusses rare forms of neoplastic disorders, such as childhood Langerhans cell histiocytosis, inflammatory myeloid neoplasia, and mesothelioma, a rare form of cancer. Eventually, the last section of the book explores rare skin diseases, for instance, epidermolysis bullosa (EB), a group of genetic skin diseases, predominantly focusing on various potential and promising treatment strategies of EB. The concluding chapter highlights the significance of stem cell-based transplant therapy of EB as well as tissue engineering-based skin substitutes that are currently available for the treatment of EB lesions.

This book is highly valuable not only for medical and allied health students but also for researchers, clinical and nurse geneticists, genetic counselors, and physician assistants. This quick reference will benefit anyone desiring a thorough knowledge pertaining to recent advances in rare diseases and their associated diagnostic and therapeutic challenges.

I would like to thank the team at IntechOpen, including Author Service Manager Mia Vulovic and Commissioning Editors Anja Filipovic and Ana Simic, for providing excellent support throughout the preparation of this book; they were remarkably patient. Finally, I dedicate this to my best friend Dr. Abhilasha Gupta and her daughter Ananya Gupta, a voracious reader and budding scientist who always puts a smile on my face.

Mani T. Valarmathi, MD, Ph.D.
Clinical Molecular Diagnostic Laboratory,
Religen Inc. | A Life Science Company,
Plymouth Meeting,
Pennsylvania, USA

Section 1

Rare Diseases Genomics and Precision Medicine

Chapter 1

Introductory Chapter: Rare Diseases - Ending the Diagnostic Odyssey and Beginning the Therapeutic Odyssey

Mani T. Valarmathi

1. Introduction

Rare disease is any disease or condition that affects a small percentage of the population. For instance, in the United States, a rare disease is defined as a condition that affects fewer than 200 000 people, whereas in Europe, a disease is considered rare when it affects less than 1 in 2000 people within the general population. Thus, a rare disease is a health condition that affects small number of people compared with other prevalent diseases in the general population [1]. However, specific issues are raised with respect to their rarity. This implies that a disease can be rare in one region, but common in another region, for example, thalassemias, a heterogeneous group of genetic disorders of blood that reduces the production of functional hemoglobin (the protein in red blood cells that carries oxygen). Thalassemia is rare in Northern Europe but more common in the Mediterranean region as well in South and South-East Asia.

Since rare diseases are numerous, heterogeneous in nature, and geographically disparate, rare diseases are an emerging global public health priority. Until now, between 6000 to 8000 distinct rare diseases have been discovered, and new rare diseases are reported constantly in the medical literature [1]. In general, rare diseases affect more than 25 million people in the United States alone, 30 million people in the European Union, and more than 400 million people Worldwide. Generally, 72% of rare diseases are genetic origin and almost 70% of rare diseases are exclusively of pediatric onset, according to the Orphanet, a publicly available epidemiological database that contains information on 6172 unique rare diseases [2].

When of genetic origin, rare disease can be inherited, with several other affected family members, following different modes of inheritance; or they may arise in sporadic, with no other affected family members; or may occur due to *de novo* chance mutations in candidate genes. For several rare conditions, on the one hand, the signs of disease could be observed prior to or during delivery or in childhood, as in the case of achondroplasia, osteogenesis imperfecta (OI, brittle bone disease), spinal muscular atrophy (SMA), or Rett syndrome (RTT). On the other hand, the initial presentation of rare diseases can be observed only during adulthood, as in the case of Huntington's disease (HD, Huntington's Chorea), amyotrophic lateral sclerosis (ALS, Lou Gehrig's disease), Crohn's disease (IBD, inflammatory bowel disease), or Charcot–Marie–Tooth Disease (CMT, hereditary motor and sensory neuropathies). While in essence all genetic diseases are rare diseases, not all rare diseases are of genetic diseases. This indicates that there are

IntechOpen

also rare forms of non-genetic rare diseases including certain types of autoimmune diseases and rare cancers, such as systemic lupus erythematosus (SLE) and Kaposi sarcoma (KS), respectively. As well as maladies caused by infectious or toxic agents.

2. Evolving challenges and next frontiers

Rare diseases are often complex, may involve chronic illness, disability, and often premature death. As well they are characterized by a remarkably diverse set of symptoms; and relatively common symptoms can mask the underlying rare diseases, leading to frequent misdiagnosis. Symptoms can vary not only from one rare disease to another rare disease but also from one patient to another patient suffering from the same rare disease; even occasionally, the symptoms can differ from a family member to a relative with the same genetic change. At present, a few hundred rare diseases have any available treatments, in most cases, neither a cure nor highly effective treatment is available.

Due to their rarity, patients suffering from rare disease often face certain common problems and challenges, such as delay in getting a correct diagnosis; lack of information and/or scientific knowledge on their own disease; lack of appropriate healthcare; as well as difficulties and inequities in accessing treatment and care. The other lingering obstacles in developing treatment, such as safe and effective drugs and biological products for rare diseases, are due to difficulties in diagnosis; small numbers and geographically dispersed patients and scientific experts; a lack of data from natural history studies; missing biomarkers to support the clinical development of new therapeutics; as well a perception of high economic risk in developing drugs that would serve either a relatively small population with a rare disease or a larger population suffering from a common disease that primarily affects developing countries.

Understandably, nearly all rare disease patients, including their families, have endured the consequence of the so-called diagnostic odyssey, i.e., a period that encompasses from the initial disease recognition or symptom onset to the date of a definitive diagnosis, involving a battery of tests and multiple clinical visits and/or referrals, sometimes for several years, all with the hope of identifying the etiology of their disease. For more than twenty-five percent of rare disease patients, on an average it takes five years before they could be assigned a definite genetic diagnosis. Besides, some people will remain undiagnosed for their entire life.

The methodology of genetic testing of rare diseases depends critically on the exactness of the following three questions, considering β-thalassemia as an example: (1) whether the patient harbors the *specific disease causing variant* in the *specific gene*, for instance, in the case of β-thalassemia, 80% of all mutations in Greek Cypriots are c.93-21G>A; or (2) whether the patient harbors *any variant* in the β-thalassemia gene; or (3) whether the patient harbors *any variant* in *any gene* that would be responsible for his or her medical condition. Each of the above three questions can be addressed by employing methods that can detect: (1) specific sequence changes in the candidate gene; or (2) sequencing each exon of the candidate gene, probably by Sanger sequencing; or (3) by using next generation sequencing (massively parallel sequencing) technology, respectively.

With the advent of next generation sequencing platforms, such as the massively parallel/deep sequencing, has opened up the possibility of rapid identification of the disease-causing genes and genes alterations that are responsible for numerous rare diseases previously characterized only by clinical description [3]. This new technology can be harnessed in several ways for clinical molecular diagnostics purposes with its own advantages and disadvantages, for instance, one can sequence a panel of candidate genes or whole exome using exome capture kits or whole genome. The major advantage of the whole genome diagnostic sequencing compared with whole exome diagnostic sequencing is that it avoids exon capture, and this would allow changes outside coding exons to be identified routinely.

However, over the last decade, research and clinical exome sequencing efforts have been successfully harnessed at identifying not only known but missed diagnoses but also novel and newly characterized rare genetic syndromes [4, 5]. The utility of clinical exome sequencing resulted, with a diagnostic yield in the range of twenty-five to thirty percent among large and heterogeneous rare diseases cohorts [6]. Nevertheless, in more than seventy percent of patients in whom there was high degree of pre-test probability for a monogenic rare disease, exome sequencing renders no molecular diagnosis.

Despite the remarkable capability of exome sequencing to provide molecular diagnoses for rare disease patients, some pathogenic genomic variants are entirely missed by exome sequencing, for example, small insertions-deletions (indels), chromosomal rearrangements, and copy-number variants (CNVs), but these causative variants can be conclusively diagnosed by short-read genome sequencing. Similarly, rare disease secondary to pathogenic repeat expansions or rearrangements can potentially be identified or enhanced by long-read genomic sequencing. In addition, some disease mechanisms are either difficult or impossible to detect using whole exome sequencing approach, for instance, mosaicism of a pathogenic variant may not be routinely discovered by existing analytical approaches, which requires deep sequencing of multiple tissues. Even though whole genome sequencing outperforms exome sequencing, several other emerging technologies, such as transcriptome sequencing (to evaluate the functional consequence of variants) and methylation arrays (to provide insights into imprinting disorders), offer added value as adjunct diagnostic tools [7].

In general, several clinical investigations have the potential to reveal findings that are not related to the primary reason for the investigation, but that may be clinically significant. Evidently, when a patient's whole exome or whole genome sequencing is performed, it has exceptionally high potential to discover clinically relevant incidental findings. Arguably, the additional concern surrounding the whole exome and/or whole genome sequencing is how to handle the incidental findings, as they become ever more routine. In this context, the European Society of Human Genetics recommends a much more conservative approach, i.e., whenever possible, testing should be targeted to genome regions linked to the patient's indications [8–10].

Finally, the advancement of genetic medicine and precision medicine can end one odyssey and start another one, i.e., for rare disease patients, a genetic result can mark not only the end of a '*diagnostic odyssey*' but also mark the beginning of a '*therapeutic odyssey*.'

3. Conclusions

Rare diseases, even though individually rare, are collective common. Many rare conditions are not only chronically debilitating and progressive but also degenerative and life-threatening. Most do not have appropriate treatments, rendering them incurable. Consequently, drug, biologic, and device development in the case of rare disease is challenging for many reasons, including the complex biology and the lack of critical understanding of the nature course of many rare diseases. In addition, the inherently fewer population of patients with a rare disease may also cause conducting clinical trials challenging. Scientists and clinicians around the globe are working to find better ways to prevent, detect, and treat rare diseases, and to improve the quality of life of patients and their families.

Author details

Mani T. Valarmathi
Clinical Molecular Diagnostic Laboratory, Religen Inc. - A Life Science Company, Plymouth Meeting, Pennsylvania, USA

*Address all correspondence to: valarmathi64@hotmail.com

References

[1] Richter T, Nestler-Parr S, Babela R, Khan ZM, Tesoro T, Molsen E, Hughes DA. International Society for Pharmacoeconomics and Outcomes Research Rare Disease Special Interest Group. Rare Disease Terminology and Definitions-A Systematic Global Review: Report of the ISPOR Rare Disease Special Interest Group. Value Health. 2015 Sep;18(6):906-914. doi: 10.1016/j.jval.2015.05.008. Epub 2015 Aug 18. PMID: 26409619.

[2] Nguengang Wakap S, Lambert DM, Olry A, Rodwell C, Gueydan C, Lanneau V, Murphy D, Le Cam Y, Rath A. Estimating cumulative point prevalence of rare diseases: analysis of the Orphanet database. Eur J Hum Genet. 2020 Feb;28(2):165-173. doi: 10.1038/s41431-019-0508-0. Epub 2019 Sep 16. PMID: 31527858; PMCID: PMC6974615.

[3] Goodwin S, McPherson JD, McCombie WR. Coming of age: ten years of next-generation sequencing technologies. Nat Rev Genet. 2016 May 17;17(6):333-351. doi: 10.1038/nrg.2016.49. PMID: 27184599.

[4] Boycott KM, Rath A, Chong JX, Hartley T, Alkuraya FS, Baynam G, Brookes AJ, Brudno M, Carracedo A, den Dunnen JT, Dyke SOM, Estivill X, Goldblatt J, Gonthier C, Groft SC, Gut I, Hamosh A, Hieter P, Höhn S, Hurles ME, Kaufmann P, Knoppers BM, Krischer JP, Macek M Jr, Matthijs G, Olry A, Parker S, Paschall J, Philippakis AA, Rehm HL, Robinson PN, Sham PC, Stefanov R, Taruscio D, Unni D, Vanstone MR, Zhang F, Brunner H, Bamshad MJ, Lochmüller H. International Cooperation to Enable the Diagnosis of All Rare Genetic Diseases. Am J Hum Genet. 2017 May 4;100(5):695-705. doi: 10.1016/j.ajhg.2017.04.003. PMID: 28475856; PMCID: PMC5420351.

[5] Tabor HK, Goldenberg A. What Precision Medicine Can Learn from Rare Genetic Disease Research and Translation. AMA J Ethics. 2018 Sep 1;20(9):E834-E840. doi: 10.1001/amajethics.2018.834. PMID: 30242814.

[6] Clark MM, Stark Z, Farnaes L, Tan TY, White SM, Dimmock D, Kingsmore SF. Meta-analysis of the diagnostic and clinical utility of genome and exome sequencing and chromosomal microarray in children with suspected genetic diseases. NPJ Genom Med. 2018 Jul 9;3:16. doi: 10.1038/s41525-018-0053-8. PMID: 30002876; PMCID: PMC6037748.

[7] Subramanian I, Verma S, Kumar S, Jere A, Anamika K. Multi-omics Data Integration, Interpretation, and Its Application. Bioinform Biol Insights. 2020 Jan 31;14:1177932219899051. doi: 10.1177/1177932219899051. PMID: 32076369; PMCID: PMC7003173.

[8] de Wert G, Dondorp W, Clarke A, Dequeker EMC, Cordier C, Deans Z, van El CG, Fellmann F, Hastings R, Hentze S, Howard H, Macek M, Mendes A, Patch C, Rial-Sebbag E, Stefansdottir V, Cornel MC, Forzano F. European Society of Human Genetics. Opportunistic genomic screening. Recommendations of the European Society of Human Genetics. Eur J Hum Genet. 2021 Mar;29(3):365-377. doi: 10.1038/s41431-020-00758-w. Epub 2020 Nov 22. PMID: 33223530; PMCID: PMC7940405.

[9] van El CG, Cornel MC, Borry P, Hastings RJ, Fellmann F, Hodgson SV, Howard HC, Cambon-Thomsen A, Knoppers BM, Meijers-Heijboer H, Scheffer H, Tranebjaerg L, Dondorp W, de Wert GM. ESHG Public and Professional Policy Committee. Whole-genome sequencing in health care: recommendations of the European Society of Human Genetics. Eur J Hum Genet. 2013a Jun;21(6):580-584. doi: 10.1038/ejhg.2013.46. PMID: 23676617; PMCID: PMC3658192.

[10] van El CG, Dondorp WJ, de Wert GM, Cornel MC. Call for prudence in whole-genome testing. Science. 2013b Aug 30;341(6149):958-959. doi: 10.1126/science.341.6149.958-b. PMID: 23990543.

Section 2

Rare Immune System Diseases

Chapter 2

Felty's Syndrome

Vadim Gorodetskiy

Abstract

Felty's syndrome (FS) is an uncommon subset of seropositive rheumatoid arthritis (RA) complicated by neutropenia with or without splenomegaly. The pathogenesis of neutropenia in FS is still not fully understood, but it is believed that the principal cause is neutrophil survival defect. Autoantibodies against peptidylarginine deiminase type 4 deiminated histones, glucose-6-phosphate isomerase, and eukaryotic elongation factor 1A-1 antigen may contribute to neutropenia development in FS patients. Splenic histology in FS shows non-specific findings and spleen size do not correlate with neutropenia. Cases of T-cell large granular lymphocytic leukemia with low tumor burden in blood and concomitant RA are clinically indistinguishable from FS and present a diagnostic challenge. Examination of T-cell clonality, mutations in signal transducer and activator of transcription 3 gene, and the number of large granular lymphocytes in the blood can establish a correct diagnosis. Optimal approaches to therapy for FS have not been developed, but the use of rituximab seems promising. In this chapter, the epidemiology, pathogenesis, clinical manifestations, differential diagnosis, and treatment options for FS are discussed.

Keywords: Felty's syndrome, rheumatoid arthritis, neutropenia, splenomegaly, large granular lymphocyte leukemia

1. Introduction

In 1924, at Johns Hopkins Hospital, American physician Augustus Felty described five unusual cases with features of chronic arthritis, splenomegaly, and striking leukopenia [1]. In 1932, the eponym "Felty's syndrome (FS)" was first used by Hanrahan and Miller to describe these cases [2]. Currently, FS is considered an uncommon subset of seropositive rheumatoid arthritis (RA) complicated by neutropenia and splenomegaly [3]. Although splenomegaly represents one characteristic of the triad that defines FS, it is not an absolute requirement of FS diagnosis [4, 5]. T-cell large granular lymphocyte (T-LGL) leukemia in the setting of RA is the condition most likely to be confused with FS. Studies on FS should be considered with the caveat that almost all were performed without a study of T-cell clonality and, therefore, could include cases of RA-associated T-LGL leukemia (see "Diagnosis and differential diagnosis").

2. Epidemiology

About 1% to 3% of patients with RA develop FS [6]. However, with the evolution of RA pharmacotherapy, the frequency of FS has decreased substantially [7]. The mean age of the patients is 60 years, with a 1.5:1 female to male ratio [8].

3. Pathogenesis

There is firm evidence that the HLA-DRB1*04 genotype is a risk factor for FS development [9]. The exact pathophysiological mechanisms leading to development of neutropenia and splenomegaly in FS are unknown. It is believed, though, that neutrophil survival defect is the main cause of neutropenia [8, 10]. Several auto-antibodies have been found in the serum of FS patients with higher frequency or at higher titers in comparison with seropositive RA patients without FS, which may contribute to neutropenia development, including:

- autoantibodies to H3, H4, and H2A histones deiminated by peptidylarginine deiminase type 4 [11];
- autoantibodies against glucose-6-phosphate isomerase [12];
- autoantibodies against eukaryotic elongation factor 1A-1 antigen [13];
- circulating immune complexes [14].

Autoantibodies against granulocyte colony-stimulating factor (G-CSF) were found in 73% patients with FS [15]. However, given that, in most cases, bone marrow in FS reveals normal myeloid cellularity or myeloid hyperplasia with increased granulopoiesis, relative excess of immature forms, and apparent lack of mature myeloid elements [8], the pathogenetic significance of anti-G-CSF antibodies in neutropenia development in patients with FS is unclear.

Some researchers question the significance of spleen sequestration/destruction in neutropenia pathogenesis [8]. However, neutrophils are found in periarteriolar lymphoid sheaths of the spleen even in patients with severe neutropenia [16]. In addition, removal of the spleen leads to restoration of normal neutrophil counts in most patients with FS.

4. Clinical manifestations

Clinical manifestations of FS and the frequency of signs/symptoms based on literature data [5, 14, 17–19] are presented in **Table 1**.

FS usually develops 10–15 years after RA presentation [14, 20], but in rare instances, neutropenia and splenomegaly may precede an arthritis history (non-articular Felty's syndrome) [21–24].

The erosive process in FS is typically severe, but this is related to the duration of RA before the onset of neutropenia and splenomegaly [6]. RA with FS is associated with more frequent and severe extra-articular manifestations than RA without FS [14, 20]. Rheumatoid factor (RF) and anti-cyclic citrullinated peptide (anti-CCP) antibodies are associated with severe extra-articular manifestations in patients with RA [25]. This is consistent with the finding that the vast majority of patients with FS have high titers of RF [14]. In our cohort of 25 patients with FS with a median duration of RA prior to FS diagnosis of 7 years, erosive arthritis at the time of FS diagnosis was detected in 77% of the patients. RF was within the normal range in only two cases, but the anti-CCP titers in these patients were highly positive [26].

Neutropenia (absolute neutrophil count of less than 1.500–2.000/μL) without a clearly identified cause is required, by definition, for the FS diagnosis. Neutropenia can manifest as increased frequency and severity of bacterial infections. However, despite reduced absolute neutrophil counts, patients with FS can remain free of infectious complications for extended periods of time.

Signs/symptoms	Frequency (%)
Major	
Rheumatoid arthritis	100
Neutropenia	100
Splenomegaly	90
Minor	
Rheumatoid nodules	53–82
Leg ulcers	15–41
Skin pigmentation	5–29
Hepatomegaly/portal hypertension	5–68
Serositis	0–22
Lymphadenopathy	0–34
Neuropathy	11–17
Episcleritis	0–8

Table 1.
Clinical manifestations of Felty's syndrome and the frequency of signs/symptoms.

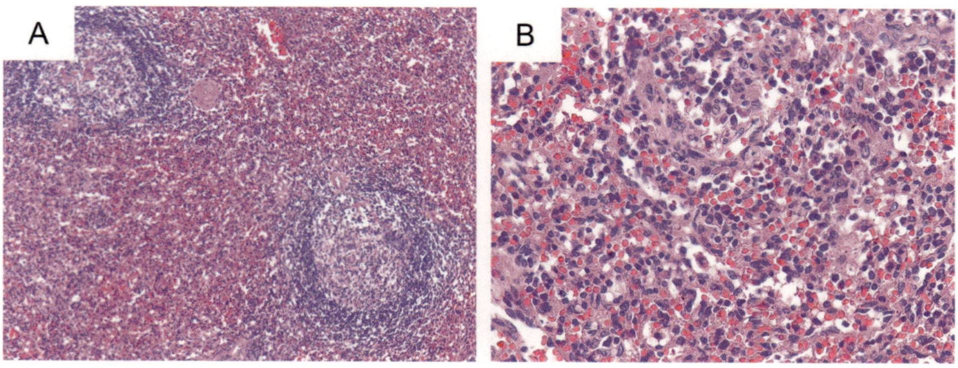

Figure 1.
Spleen histological examination in a patient with Felty's syndrome. (A) The spleen shows preservation of the white pulp with prominent germinal centers and lymphocytic infiltration of the red pulp (H&E, ×100). (B) Lymphocytes infiltrate both cords and sinusoids. The infiltration is more prominent within the splenic cords (H&E, ×400).

Splenomegaly is present in over 90% of patients with FS, but the spleen size does not correlate with neutropenia [14, 17, 19]. Splenic histology in FS shows non-specific findings (**Figure 1**). The red pulp shows expanded sinuses as well as the pulp cords, and an increased number of macrophages and plasma cells. The white pulp follicles are usually hyperplastic [18, 27, 28]. It is possible that portal hypertension secondary to nodular regenerative hyperplasia of the liver contributes to spleen enlargement in some patients with FS [29].

5. Diagnosis and differential diagnosis

FS should be suspected in a patient with RA, unexplained neutropenia, and splenomegaly. There is a wide range of pathologies in patients with RA that can manifest with neutropenia with or without splenomegaly. FS is a clinical diagnosis, and there is no specific single diagnostic test to confirm or exclude it; therefore, FS is essentially a diagnosis of exclusion.

Neutropenia caused by drug therapy (drug-induced neutropenia) should be ruled out first. The most important treatment of drug-induced neutropenia is to withdraw the causative drug. The average time for full recovery of the neutrophil count is 9 days (range, 9–24 days) [30]. Methotrexate, cyclophosphamide, azathioprine, sulfasalazine, leflunomide, tocilizumab, tumor necrosis factor (TNF)-alpha antagonists, antimalarial medications, analgesics, and nonsteroidal anti-inflammatory drugs are the most common causes of drug-induced neutropenia in patients with RA [28]. It is important to keep in mind that unlike with other drugs, rituximab-induced neutropenia occurs after a median period of 4.5 months (range, 3–6.5 months) after the last rituximab infusion [31].

T-LGL leukemia is a rare type of mature T-cell neoplasm characterized by the clonal expansion of large granular lymphocytes (LGLs) and, in most cases, has indolent clinical course. Typical features of T-LGL leukemia include the increase in the number of peripheral blood LGLs, cytopenia (most commonly neutropenia), and variable splenomegaly. A peculiar feature of T-LGL leukemia is its association with RA, which occurs in 17–28% of patients with T-LGL leukemia [32, 33]. Historically, a definitive diagnosis of T-LGL leukemia required the increase in the number of LGLs in peripheral blood greater than 2×10^9/L, but it is now recognized that a lower count (range, $0.4–2 \times 10^9$/L) may be compatible with the diagnosis [34–36].

Cases of T-LGL leukemia in the setting of RA (RA-associated T-LGL leukemia) with low LGL count in peripheral blood and concomitant neutropenia are clinically indistinguishable from FS and diagnostically challenging. RA-associated T-LGL leukemia and FS are distinguished in clinical practice by evaluation of rearrangements of the T cell receptor (TCR) gamma and TCR beta genes in the blood and/or in the bone marrow. The monoclonal rearrangements of the TCR genes (T-cell clonality) are present in T-LGL leukemia but not in FS (**Figure 2**) [3, 8, 37]. However,

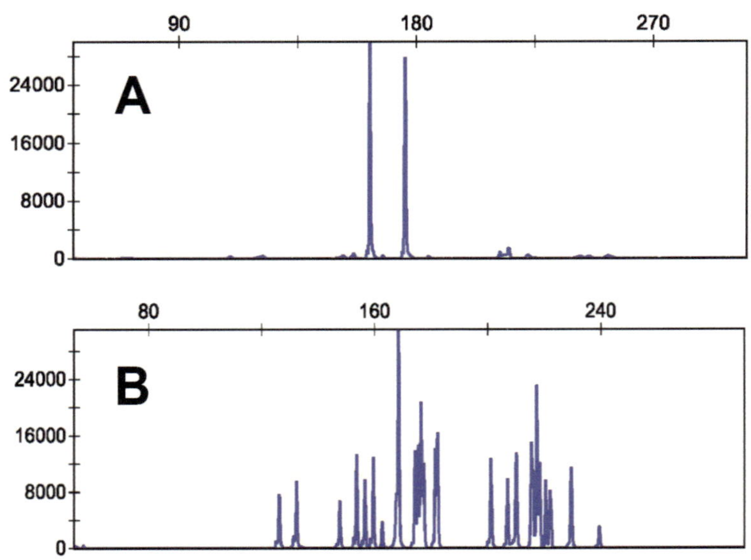

Figure 2.
Evaluation of T-cell clonality based on rearrangements of the T-cell receptor (TCR) genes. (A) TCR genes show monoclonal rearrangement in T-LGL leukemia. (B) TCR genes show polyclonal rearrangement in Felty's syndrome.

there is considerable discussion regarding the significance of dominant T-cell clones as a hallmark of T-cell malignancy because clonal populations of T-cells are observed both in healthy individuals and in exuberant reactive responses [38–43]. Activating somatic mutations in the signal transducer and activator of the transcription 3 (STAT3) gene and an increase in the number of LGLs above 2×10^9/L were detected in RA-associated T-LGL leukemia but not in FS (39% vs. 0% and 21% vs. 0%, respectively) [26]. In addition, the expression of the CD57 antigen and the aberrant (diminished or absent) expression of CD5 on cytotoxic CD3 + CD8+ T-lymphocytes are more typical for T-LGL leukemia than in the polyclonal expansion of cytotoxic T-lymphocytes in FS [26]. In contrast, it seems that the current criteria for bone marrow involvement in T-LGL leukemia do not seem to be sufficiently specific to distinguish it from FS [8, 26].

Aplastic anemia, myelodysplastic syndromes, or acute leukemia can sometimes present with isolated neutropenia. To rule out these pathologies, a bone marrow examination should be considered. In rare cases, cirrhosis, amyloidosis, lymphomas involving spleen, sarcoidosis, or infections can lead to splenomegaly in patients with RA.

6. Management

In two earlier analyzes of survival in FS, 5-year mortality ranged from 25% to 36% [5, 44]; however, recent data regarding the prognosis of FS are not available. The treatment goal in FS is a reversal of the neutropenia to prevent recurrent bacterial infections and sepsis, which is the leading cause of death in patients with FS. The treatment strategy for FS is not evidence-based because of the lack of controlled trials.

Methotrexate (MTX) is considered the first-line therapy for treatment of FS based on case reports and case series data. Low doses of MTX (up to 25 mg once a week) can improve both joint diseases and neutropenia, usually within 1–2 months.

One recent literature review supported the use of rituximab (RTX) as a second-line therapy. A sustained increase in the absolute number of neutrophils was observed in 62.5% of FS patients during the 3 months following one cycle of RTX treatment [45]. The appropriate dosing schedule of RTX for treatment of FS remains uncertain, but most often patients receive two 1000 mg doses separated by 15 days [46]. Some patients had a recurrence of neutropenia after RTX treatment, indicating that in some cases a sustained response may require maintenance therapy with RTX.

There is very limited evidence regarding the leflunomide efficacy in FS [47]. TNF-alpha inhibitors (adalimumab, ethanercept, and infliximab) are ineffective in FS [45].

Splenectomy maintained normal neutrophil counts in 80% of patients with FS [10]. However, the indications for splenectomy are now limited because of effective medications and the risk of post-splenectomy sepsis.

The results of treatment with glucocorticoids (GCs) in patients with FS are variable. GCs can provide a rapid improvement in neutrophil count by stimulating the release of mature cells from the bone marrow and mobilizing them from the marginal pool, thus, creating the effect of increasing their absolute number. However, to achieve a real clinical effect, high doses and prolonged use of GCs may be required, which increases the risk of infection in patients with FS.

G-CSF can be used for treatment of FS patients with life-threatening infections.

7. Conclusion

Although nearly 100 years have passed since the first description of FS, this pathology remains a mystery in many aspects. The pathogenetic mechanisms underlying neutropenia and spleen enlargement in these patients are poorly understood. Optimal approaches to therapy for this rare disorder have not been developed, but the use of rituximab seems promising.

Acknowledgements

I would like to thank Editage (www.editage.com) for English language editing.

Conflict of interest

The author declares no conflict of interest.

Author details

Vadim Gorodetskiy
Department of Intensive Methods of Therapy, V.A. Nasonova Research Institute of Rheumatology, Moscow, Russia

*Address all correspondence to: gorodetskiyblood@mail.ru

References

[1] Felty AR. Chronic arthritis in the adult associated with splenomegaly and leukopenia. Bull Johns Hopkins Hosp. 1924; 35:16-20

[2] Hanrahan EM, Miller SR. Effect of splenectomy in Felty's syndrome. JAMA. 1932; 99:1247-1252

[3] Balint GP, Balint PV. Felty's syndrome. Best Pract Res Clin Rheumatol. 2004;18,631-645. DOI:10.1016/j.berh.2004.05.002

[4] Spivak JL. Felty's syndrome: an analytical review. Johns Hopkins Med J. 1977;141:156-162

[5] Campion G, Maddison PJ, Goulding N, James I, Ahern MJ, Watt I, Sansom D. The Felty syndrome: a case-matched study of clinical manifestations and outcome, serologic features, and immunogenetic associations. Medicine (Baltimore). 1990;69:69-80

[6] Sibley JT, Haga M, Visram DA, Mitchell DM. The clinical course of Felty's syndrome compared to matched controls. J. Rheumatol. 1991;18:1163-1167

[7] Bartels CM, Bell CL, Shinki K, Rosenthal A, Bridges AJ. Changing trends in serious extra-articular manifestations of rheumatoid arthritis among United State veterans over 20 years. Rheumatology (Oxford). 2010;49:1670-1675. DOI: 10.1093/rheumatology/keq135

[8] Burks EJ, Loughran TP Jr. Pathogenesis of neutropenia in large granular lymphocyte leukemia and Felty syndrome. Blood Rev. 2006;20:245-266. DOI: 10.1016/j.blre.2006.01.003

[9] Turesson C, Schaid DJ, Weyand CM, Jacobsson LT, Goronzy JJ, PeterssonIF,SturfeltG,Nyhäll-WåhlinBM, Truedsson L, Dechant SA, Matteson EL. The impact of HLA-DRB1 genes on extra-articular disease manifestations in rheumatoid arthritis. Arthritis Res Ther. 2005;7:R1386–R1393. DOI: 10.1186/ar1837

[10] Rashba EJ, Rowe JM, Packman CH. Treatment of the neutropenia of Felty syndrome. Blood Rev. 1996;10:177-184. DOI: 10.1016/s0268-960x(96)90024-7

[11] Dwivedi N, Upadhyay J, Neeli I, Khan S, Pattanaik D, Myers L, Kirou KA, Hellmich B, Knuckley B, Thompson PR, Crow MK, Mikuls TR, Csernok E, Radic M. Felty's syndrome autoantibodies bind to deiminated histones and neutrophil extracellular chromatin traps. Arthritis Rheum. 2012;64:982-992. DOI: 10.1002/art.33432

[12] van Gaalen FA, Toes RE, Ditzel HJ, Schaller M, Breedveld FC, Verweij CL, Huizinga TW. Association of autoantibodies to glucose-6-phosphate isomerase with extraarticular complications in rheumatoid arthritis. Arthritis Rheum. 2004;50:395-399. DOI: 10.1002/art.20028

[13] Ditzel HJ, Masaki Y, Nielsen H, Farnaes L, Burton DR. Cloning and expression of a novel human antibody-antigen pair associated with Felty's syndrome. Proc Natl Acad Sci U S A. 2000;97:9234-9239. DOI: 10.1073/pnas.97.16.9234

[14] Goldberg J, Pinals RS. Felty syndrome. Semin Arthritis Rheum. 1980;10:52-65. DOI: 10.1016/0049-0172(80)90014-1

[15] Hellmich B, Csernok E, Schatz H, Gross WL, Schnabel A. Autoantibodies against granulocyte colony-stimulating factor in Felty's syndrome and neutropenic systemic lupus erythematosus. Arthritis Rheum.

2002;46:2384-2391. DOI: 10.1002/art.10497

[16] O'Malley DP, George TI, Orazi A, Abbondanzo SL. Benign and Reactive Conditions of Lymph Node and Spleen (Atlas of Nontumor Pathology). 1st ed. American Registry of Pathology Washington, DC in collaboration with the Armed Forces Institute of Pathology Washington, DC; 2009. p.390-391.

[17] Ruderman M, Miller LM, Pinals RS. Clinical and serologic observations on 27 patients with Felty's syndrome. Arthritis Rheum. 1968;11:377-384. DOI: 10.1002/art.1780110302

[18] Barnes CG, Turnbull AL, Vernon-Roberts B. Felty's syndrome. A clinical and pathological survey of 21 patients and their response to treatment. Ann Rheum Dis. 1971;30:359-374. DOI: 10.1136/ard.30.4.359

[19] Sienknecht CW, Urowitz MB, Pruzanski W, Stein HB. Felty's syndrome. Clinical and serological analysis of 34 cases. Ann Rheum Dis. 1977;36:500-507. DOI: 10.1136/ard.36.6.500

[20] Rosenstein ED, Kramer N. Felty's and pseudo-Felty's syndromes. Semin Arthritis Rheum. 1991;2:129-142. DOI: 10.1016/0049-0172(91)90002-h

[21] Bradley JD, Pinals RS. Felty's syndrome presenting without arthritis. Clin Exp Rheumatol. 1983;1:257-259

[22] Rozin A, Hoffman R, Hayek T, Balbir-Gurman A. Felty's syndrome without rheumatoid arthritis? Clin Rheumatol. 2013;32:701-704. DOI: 10.1007/s10067-012-2157-3

[23] Jain T, Mittal C, Sengupta R, Rubin B. Non-articular Felty's syndrome: An uncommon diagnosis. Neth J Med. 2015;73:435-436

[24] Aslam F, Cheema RS, Feinstein M, Chang-Miller A. Neutropaenia and splenomegaly without arthritis: think rheumatoid arthritis. BMJ Case Rep. 2018;2018:bcr2018225359. DOI: 10.1136/bcr-2018-225359

[25] Turesson C, Jacobsson LT, Sturfelt G, Matteson EL, Mathsson L, Rönnelid J. Rheumatoid factor and antibodies to cyclic citrullinated peptides are associated with severe extra-articular manifestations in rheumatoid arthritis. Ann Rheum Dis. 2007;66:59-64. DOI: 10.1136/ard.2006.054445

[26] Gorodetskiy VR, Sidorova YV, Kupryshina NA, Vasilyev VI, Probatova NA, Ryzhikova NV, Sudarikov AB. Analysis of a single-institution cohort of patients with Felty's syndrome and T-cell large granular lymphocytic leukemia in the setting of rheumatoid arthritis. Rheumatol Int. 2021;41:147-156. doi: 10.1007/s00296-020-04757-4

[27] van Krieken JH, Breedveld FC, te Velde J. The spleen in Felty's syndrome: a histological, morphometrical, and immunohistochemical study. Eur J Haematol. 1988;40:58-64. DOI: 10.1111/j.1600-0609.1988.tb00797.x

[28] Lazaro E, Morel J. Management of neutropenia in patients with rheumatoid arthritis. Joint Bone Spine. 2015;82:235-239. DOI: 10.1016/j.jbspin.2015.01.005

[29] Stock H, Kadry Z, Smith JP. Surgical management of portal hypertension in Felty's syndrome: A case report and literature review. J Hepatol. 2009;50:831-835. DOI: 10.1016/j.jhep.2008.10.035

[30] Pick AM, Nystrom KK. Nonchemotherapy Drug-Induced Neutropenia and Agranulocytosis: Could Medications be the Culprit? Journal of Pharmacy Practice. 2014;27:447-452. DOI:10.1177/0897190014546115

[31] Salmon JH, Cacoub P, Combe B, Sibilia J, Pallot-Prades B, Fain O, Cantagrel A, Dougados M, Andres E, Meyer O, Carli P, Pertuiset E, Pane I, Maurier F, Ravaud P, Mariette X, Gottenberg JE. Late-onset neutropenia after treatment with rituximab for rheumatoid arthritis and other autoimmune diseases: data from the AutoImmunity and Rituximab registry. RMD Open. 2015;1:e000034. DOI: 10.1136/rmdopen-2014-000034

[32] Loughran TP Jr. Clonal diseases of large granular lymphocytes. Blood. 1993;82:1-14

[33] Bareau B, Rey J, Hamidou M, Donadieu J, Morcet J, Reman O, Schleinitz N, Tournilhac O, Roussel M, Fest T, Lamy T. Analysis of a French cohort of patients with large granular lymphocyte leukemia: a report on 229 cases. Haematologica. 2010;95:1534-1541. DOI: 10.3324/haematol.2009.018481

[34] Semenzato G, Zambello R, Starkebaum G, Oshimi K, Loughran TP Jr. The lymphoproliferative disease of granular lymphocytes: updated criteria for diagnosis. Blood. 1997;89:256-260

[35] Moignet A, Lamy T. Latest advances in the diagnosis and treatment of large granular lymphocytic leukemia. Am Soc Clin Oncol Educ Book. 2018;38:616-625. DOI: 10.1200/EDBK_200689

[36] Cheon H, Dziewulska KH, Moosic KB, Olson KC, Gru AA, Feith DJ, Loughran TP Jr. Advances in the Diagnosis and Treatment of Large Granular Lymphocytic Leukemia. Curr Hematol Malig Rep.2020; 15:103-112. DOI: 10.1007/s11899-020-00565-6

[37] Shah A, Diehl LF, St Clair EW. T cell large granular lymphocyte leukemia associated with rheumatoid arthritis and neutropenia. Clin Immunol. 2009;132:145-152. DOI: 10.1016/j.clim.2009.03.515

[38] Posnett DN, Sinha R, Kabak S, Russo C. Clonal populations of T cells in normal elderly humans: the T cell equivalent to "benign monoclonal gammapathy". J Exp Med. 1994;179:609-618. DOI: 10.1084/jem.179.2.609

[39] Delfau-Larue MH, Laroche L, Wechsler J, Lepage E, Lahet C, Asso-Bonnet M, Bagot M, Farcet JP. Diagnostic value of dominant T-cell clones in peripheral blood in 363 patients presenting consecutively with a clinical suspicion of cutaneous lymphoma. Blood. 2000;96:2987-2992

[40] Dippel E, Klemke D, Hummel M, Stein H, Goerdt S. T-cell clonality of undetermined significance. Blood. 2001;98:247-248. DOI: 10.1182/blood.v98.1.247

[41] Bigouret V, Hoffmann T, Arlettaz L, Villard J, Colonna M, Ticheli A, Gratwohl A, Samii K, Chapuis B, Rufer N, Roosnek E. Monoclonal T-cell expansions in asymptomatic individuals and in patients with large granular leukemia consist of cytotoxic effector T cells expressing the activating CD94:NKG2C/E and NKD2D killer cell receptors. Blood. 2003;101:3198-3204. DOI: 10.1182/blood-2002-08-2408

[42] Shi M, Olteanu H, Jevremovic D, He R, Viswanatha D, Corley H, Horna P. T-cell clones of uncertain significance are highly prevalent and show close resemblance to T-cell large granular lymphocytic leukemia. Implications for laboratory diagnostics. Mod Pathol. 2020;33:2046-2057. DOI: 10.1038/s41379-020-0568-2

[43] Sidorova YV, Sychevskaya KA, Chernova NG, Julhakyan HL, Smirnova SJ, Ryzhikova NV, Gorodetskiy VR, Naumova EV, Sudarikov AB. High Incidence of Clonal CD8+ T-cell Proliferation in Non-malignant Conditions May Reduce the Significance of T-cell Clonality Assay for Differential Diagnosis in Oncohematology.

Clin Lymphoma Myeloma Leuk. 2020;20:203-208. DOI: 10.1016/j.clml.2019.12.021

[44] Thorne C, Urowitz MB. Long-term outcome in Felty's syndrome. Ann Rheum Dis. 1982;41:486-489. DOI: 10.1136/ard.41.5.486

[45] Narváez J, Domingo-Domenech E, Gómez-Vaquero C, López-Vives L, Estrada P, Aparicio M, Martín-Esteve I, Nolla JM. Biological agents in the management of Felty's syndrome: a systematic review. Semin Arthritis Rheum. 2012;41:658-668. DOI: 10.1016/j.semarthrit.2011.08.008

[46] Wang CR, Chiu YC, Chen YC. Successful treatment of refractory neutropenia in Felty's syndrome with rituximab. Scand J Rheumatol. 2018;47:340-341. DOI: 10.1080/03009742.2017.1334816

[47] Yazıcı A, Uçar A, Mehtap Ö, Gönüllü EÖ, Tamer A. Presentation of three cases followed up with a diagnosis of Felty syndrome. Eur J Rheumatol. 2014;1:120-122. DOI: 10.5152/eurjrheumatol.2014.026

Chapter 3

Löfgren's Syndrome

Shiyu Wang and Shailendra Singh

Abstract

Löfgren's syndrome presents as acute sarcoid arthritis, with a triad of hilar adenopathy, acute polyarthritis and erythema nodosum. Löfgren's syndrome is self-limited, erythema nodosum, hilar adenopathy and acute polyarthritis usually resolve within a few weeks to months, however polyarthritis can last for up to 2 years. Treatment involves symptomatic control with NSAIDs/colchicine or oral glucocorticoids until symptoms resolve, if disease is resistant to these therapies, hydroxychloroquine, methotrexate or infliximab can be used. Löfgren's syndrome is a rare presentation of sarcoidosis occurring in only about 5–10% of sarcoid patients. It is, however, important to recognize as it is the most common form of acute sarcoid arthritis and prompt treatment can prevent unnecessary prolonged discomfort for patients.

Keywords: Löfgren's Syndrome, Sarcoidosis, Polyarthritis, Hilar adenopathy, Erythema nodosum

1. Introduction

Löfgren's syndrome is an acute manifestation of sarcoidosis. Sarcoidosis is a disease characterized by noncaseating granulomas throughout multiple body systems, most commonly involving the lungs (> 90% cases), often manifesting as hilar adenopathy. A small subset of patients (~10%) will develop joints symptoms, which can manifest as either acute or chronic arthritis. Löfgren's syndrome is the most common presentation of acute sarcoid arthritis, occurring in about 5–10% of sarcoid cases, presenting as classical triad of acute polyarthritis, erythema nodosum and hilar adenopathy.

2. Epidemiology

Sarcoidosis is a disease with prevalence of about 10 to 20 per 100,000 people, it affects a wide variety of patients, but there are certain predilections and patterns for higher disease activity. Geographic area, ethnicity, gender and age seem to play important roles in incidence and presentation of disease [1, 2]. Various geographic locations have been studied, and there seems to be clustering of sarcoidosis incidence around certain geographic areas, with northern countries (such as Scandinavia) having much higher incidence than other areas [3]. Ethnicity also has a distinct pattern, with African Americans, Scandinavians, Afro Caribbeans, Irish, Puerto Rican and North Africans having highest incidence, though this seems to be affected by geographical location as well [3, 4]. There are also differences in disease presentation between different ethnicities; African Americans seem to have more severe disease presentation than Caucasians [2]. Lowest incidence occurs in Spain and Japan [3, 4]. Women are overall more affected by sarcoidosis than men, though interestingly, the age of diagnosis is almost 10 years later in women than men in many populations [3, 4]. There also seem to be difference in disease presentation between women and men, with women potentially experiencing more musculoskeletal related symptoms [3]. Sarcoidosis incidence also increases with family history of the disease; studies have shown that alleles on short arm of chromosome 6 seem to confer increased risk (HLA DR 11, 12, 14, 15, 17) or protection (HLA DRI, DR4) from disease [5].

Löfgren's syndrome follows many of the same epidemiologic trends of sarcoidosis. It affects women more than men, with Scandinavian ethnicity having the highest incidence [6, 7]. There also seems to be a temporal clustering of incidence, with rates highest in the months from March to July [6]. The age of onset was, however; significantly lower for Löfgren's syndrome than sarcodosis, at 39 years old versus 47 years old [7]. There also are differences between sexes in regards to presentation, women are more likely to present with erythema nodosum, whereas men are more likely to have inflammation or arthritis of ankles without erythema nodosum [8]. Various genetic factors and alleles have been associated with Löfgren's syndrome, some protective and leading to better outcomes (HLA DQB1*0201, DRB1*03) while others are associated with more severe disease and worse outcomes (CCR2, HLA DQ2, DR3) [6, 9–12].

3. Etiology

The etiology of sarcoidosis, and by extension Löfgren's syndrome, is poorly understood. Granulomatous inflammation leads to eventual noncaseating granulomas in various organs. Formation of granulomas is due to exaggerated cell mediated immune response to antigens. The exact antigen(s) that stimulate sarcoidosis is unclear at this point in time. Many studies analyzing a large number of patients have not found one factor(s) that clearly causes sarcoidosis [13], possibly due to there being many different underlying causes of sacroidosis that leads to similar presentations. Some of the possible etiologies explored to date are environmental exposures and infectious agents.

3.1 Environmental exposure

Certain chemical elements (Beryllium, Zirconium, Aluminum) have been shown to cause graulomatous disease in lungs of patients with occupational exposure to these elements, while they themselves do not cause sarcoidosis, various studies have investigated if other environmental exposures could [14–16]. Specifically, rescue workers exposed to World Trade Center dust and debris developed new onset sarcoidosis, possible due to exposure to a yet unknown component of the dust [17].

3.2 Infectious agent

Mycobacterium and Propionibacteria have been studied as possible causes of sarcoidosis [18, 19]. *Mycobacterium tuberculosis* causes granulmatous caseations similar to those seen in sarcoidosis, and there have been *Mycobacterium tuberculosis* components found in sacroidosis tissue [20]. Propionibacteria acnes have also been found in lymph nodes of sarcoidosis patients [19]. Despite these findings, there has been no casual relationship found between these infectious agents and sacroidosis. Further evidence to support an infectious etiology of sarcoidosis is that transplantations of various organs have been shown to induce sarcoidosis in recipient [21–23].

4. Pathophysiology

The pathophysiology of sarcoidosis, and by extension Löfgren's syndrome, involves activation of immune cells by as of yet unknown antigen(s). While the end result is graumloma formation, there are quite a few steps before this stage.

Antigen presenting cells (APCs), either macrophages or dendritic cells, phagocytose the as of yet unknown antigen(s), and then presents this antigen(s) to Helper CD4+ T cells. These Helper T cells then expresses various inflammatory cytokines including: interferon-gamma, Tumor necrosis factor (TNF), interleukin (IL)-2, IL-17 and IL-22 [24]. IL-17 recruits T Helper 17 (Th17) cells which then produce even more inflammatory cytokines, primarily interferon-gamma [25]. All these inflammatory mediators cause fusion of APCs into multinucleated giant cells, the APCs and multinucleated giant cells then cluster to form granulomas.

This process seems to occur most prominent and commonly in the lungs, with alveolar macrophages often the first to aggregate to form granulomas. This process can occur in other areas of the body, as evidence by up to 30% of patient experiencing extrapulmonary symptoms (**Figure 1**) [26].

4.1 Erythema Nodosum and acute polyarthritis

In Löfgren's syndrome, in addition to pulmonary granolumas (represented as hilar adenopathy), there are also manifestations of erythema nodosum and acute polyarthritis. Erythema nodosum is caused by delayed type hypersensitivity reaction from exposure to antigens. Its exact pathophysiology is not fully understood, but may be due to immune complex deposition in venules of subcutaneous

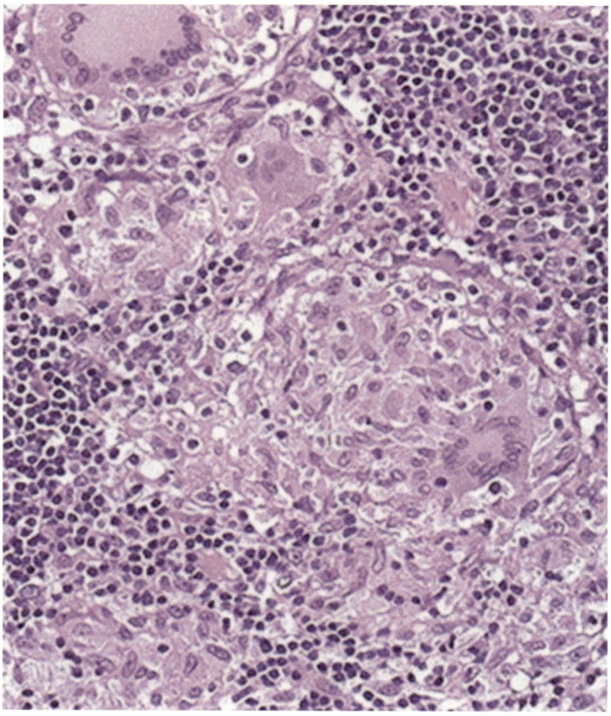

Figure 1.
Non-caseating granuloma (Samir at the English-language Wikipedia, CC BY-SA 3.0 <http://creativecommons.org/licenses/by-sa/3.0/>, via Wikimedia Commons).

fat, inciting an inflammatory reaction and granuloma formation [27]. Acute polyarthritis also has poorly understood pathogenesis, but may be due increased inflammatory milieu within the body, leading to transient inflammatory arthritis.

5. Presentation

Löfgren's syndrome presents classically as a triad of hilar lympadenopathy, erythema nodosum and acute polyarthritis. Often constitutional symptoms occur concurrently with the above triad, most commonly manifesting as fever, fatigue and malaise. Age of onset is generally under or around 40 years of age. More rare symptoms include uveitis along with blurry vision and light sensitivity [28]. There is variability in presentation between different sexes [8].

5.1 Hilar lymphadenopathy

Hilar lyphadenopathy is a classic finding of pulmonary sarcoidosis, making it ubiquitous in Löfgren's syndrome. It is a radiographic term for enlarged mediastinal lymph nodes, most often those surrounding the pulmonary hila or root of the lung, where the lungs connect to the trachea and heart. Often the enlargement is bilateral and symmetric, though the right side may be slightly more prominent. Chest radiograph is required for definitive diagnosis, and there are five stages, as discussed below. These stages do not represent disease activity, just anatomical findings on chest radiography [29]. Generally, hilar lympadenopathy will regress within 1 year [30]. Though not exclusively caused by bilateral hilar lympadenopathy, respiratory symptoms are often the first presentation that prompts obtaining a chest radiograph, where hilar lymphadenopathy is first discovered in a patient. These respiratory symptoms most commonly are coughing, dyspnea and chest pain (**Table 1** and **Figures 2** and **3**).

5.2 Erythema Nodosum

Erythema nodosum presents as erythematous, tender, immobile nodules that are elevated and can join to form a plaque. Most commonly, they present on shins in Löfgren's syndrome, though they can also appear on head and neck regions as well. These nodules are caused by subcutaneous inflammation, and are frequently accompanied by fevers and take a few days to develop. Spontaneous resolution typically occurs within eight weeks without scarring. There may be hyperpigmentation after resolution, but this is rare [27]. Relapsing erythema nodosum

Stages of Pulmonary Sarcoidosis	Features
Stage 0	Normal chest radiograph
Stage I	Bilateral hilar lymphadenopathy
Stage II	Bilateral hilar lymphadenopathy + Diffuse infiltrative lung damage
Stage III	Diffuse infiltrative lung damage
Stage IV	Lung fibrosis[1]

[1]*The Foundations in Diagnostic Pathology Series, Pulmonary Pathology – Chapter 17.*

Table 1.
Stages of pulmonary sarcoidosis.

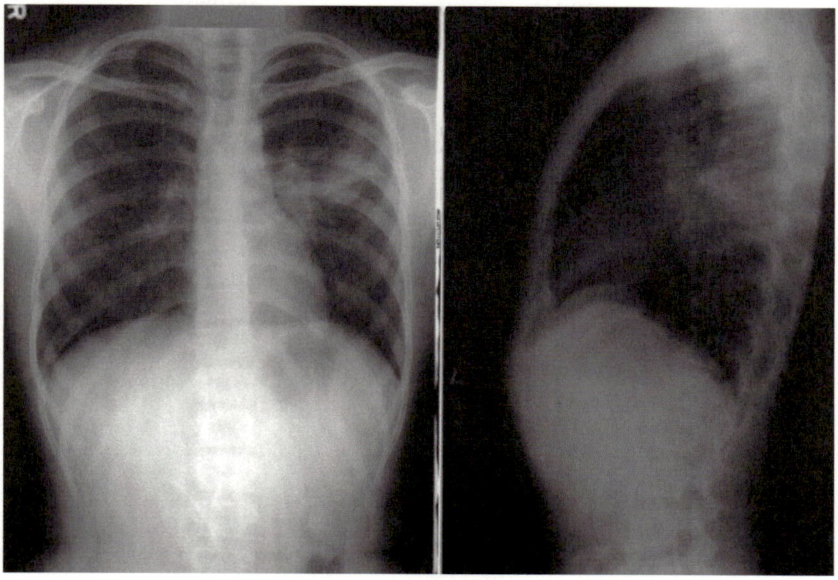

Figure 2.
Anterior–posterior and lateral chest radiograph of bilateral hilar lymphadenopathy (image courtesy of H. Bruce Dull, MD).

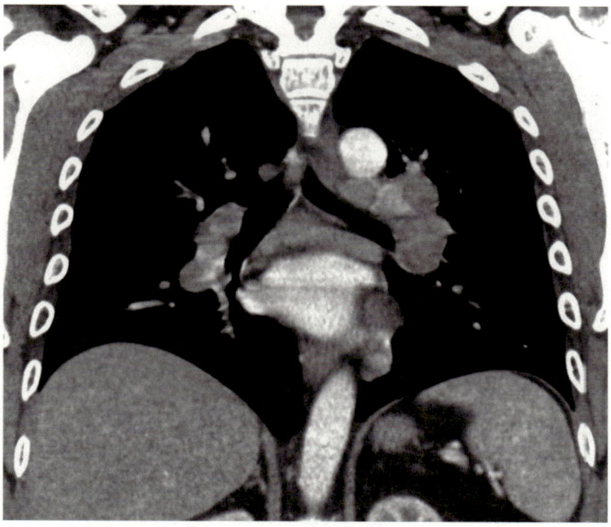

Figure 3.
Computed tomography of bilateral hilar lymphadenopathy (by James Heilman, MD - Own work, CC BY-SA 4.0, https://commons.wikimedia.org/w/index.php?curid=49068286).

can develop; this represents poor control or failure of treatment of underlying chronic condition. Erythema nodosum is also more commonly seen in women with Löfgren's syndrome, whereas men can have acute polyarthritis with no erythema nodosum (**Figure 4**) [8].

5.3 Acute polyarthritis

Acute polyarthritis in Löfgren's syndrome is typically symmetrical and oligoarticular (affecting 2 to 4 joints) initially. Most often, it involves the ankles bilaterally and then starts to affects other joints of the lower extremities such as knees and

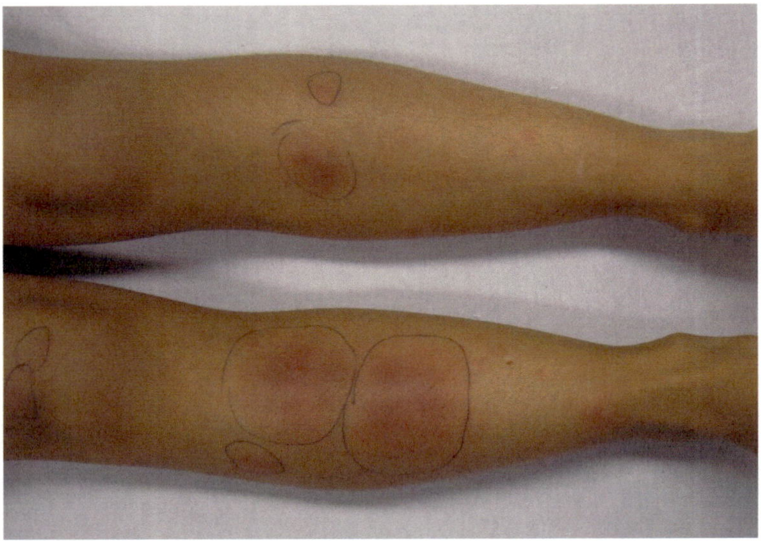

Figure 4.
Erythema nodosum of lower extremities (by James Heilman, MD - Own work, CC BY-SA 3.0, https://commons.wikimedia.org/w/index.php?curid=11520780).

can also affect wrists and elbow joints as well. Bilateral ankle arthritis seems to be the most common initial manifestation of acute polyarthritis. Rarely, small joints of hands bilaterally can be involved [30]. Arthritis generally resolves within a few months, though it can persist up to 2 years, even with treatment. Cases of recurrent arthritis after treatment have also been described [31]. Men present with acute polyarthritis more commonly [8].

6. Evaluation and diagnosis

There are no definitive test or classification criteria for Löfgren's syndrome, and though the classic triad of hilar lympadenopathy, erythema nodosum and acute polyarthritis are highly specific (> 95%), there are instances where not all components are presents in patients with Löfgren's syndrome [32]. For successful evaluation of a patient with Löfgren's syndrome, an accurate and detail history and physical must first be performed, usually followed up with a chest radiograph to confirm diagnosis. Biopsies may be indicated for definitive diagnosis of sarcoidosis if chest radiograph or other forms of imaging are inconclusive. Laboratory testing is generally not required.

6.1 History and physical exam

A detailed and accurate history and physical exam is essential for evaluation and diagnosis of Löfgren's syndrome. Chronicity and specificity symptoms need to be elucidated and investigated. Importantly, history should uncover onset and location of acute polyarthritis, and whether there has been any migration of arthritis. Underlying arthritis or arthralgias should also be clarified, to ensure that the acute polyarthritis is indeed new and acute in nature, not a continuation of previous disease. Constitutional symptoms should also be inquired about, as acute onset of fever very often accompanies both the acute polyarthritis and development of erythema nodosum. Ask about respiratory symptoms, as they can be the first sign of previously unknown hilar lymphadenopathy. Keep in mind the differences in presentation between men and women, as women may not have presentation of acute polyarthritis and just erythema nodosum, whereas men may not present with erythema nodosum.

Physical exam should include detailed examination of lower extremities, neck and head regions for erythema nodosum. Joint examination of lower extremities as well as hands, wrists and elbows should be performed to see if there is pain, tenderness, swelling, redness and heat. Monitoring temperature can also be useful in determining if there is accompanying fever with these symptoms. A detailed cardiac, pulmonary and abdominal exam should be performed as hilar adenopathy and sarcoidosis in general can cause various manifestations and physical changes in these areas.

6.2 Chest radiography

Chest radiography should be obtained at least once on all patients suspected with Löfgren's syndrome, it is an essential step to establishing if there his hilar lymphadenopathy. Section 5.1 describes findings and diagnostic criteria for hilar lymphadenopathy on chest radiograph. If chest radiography is inconclusive, high resolution computed tomography (HRCT) scan can be performed, and provides more detailed imaging and analysis of mesiatinum, able to identify in more detail the precise location and extent of lympadenopathy [33]. HRCT is not routinely recommended for evaluation and diagnosis of Löfgren's syndrome.

6.3 Biopsies

Biopsies are generally limited to cases of Löfgren's syndrome where HRCT or other imaging modalities cannot detect sarcoidosis, and/or disease is refractory to treatment or deviates from expected course. It is utilized to definitively obtain tissue samples that confirm diagnosis of sarcoidosis. Generally, bronchoalveolar lavage (BAL) is performed with endobronchial or transbronchial biopsies, endobronchial ultrasound (EBUS) biopsy can also be used for various positions and angles to attempt a needle aspiration biopsy of lympadenopathy. A triad of CD4 to CD8 cell ratio > 4, lymphocyte percentage > 16% and presence of noncaseating granulomas has 100% positive predictive value and 81% negative predictive value for diagnosis of sarcoidosis [34].

6.4 Laboratory and genetic testing

Laboratory testing is generally not required for evaluation and diagnosis of Löfgren's syndrome. Many laboratory testing is non-specific and do not provide additional value. Exceptions may include angiotensin-converting enzyme (ACE) and ionized calcium. Studies have shown that patients with elevated ACE and ionized calcium may have increased risk for prolonged arthritis [35]. Tuberculosis skin or interferon-gamma testing should be performed at least once on patients suspected with Löfgren's syndrome to rule out tuberculosis, which can mimic erythema nodosum as well as hilar adenopathy.

Genetic testing is not required for evaluation and diagnosis of Löfgren's syndrome. Though some alleles and genes have been associated with Löfgren's syndrome, they are more for academic research purposes rather than to diagnose the disease. Associations include: HLA DQB1*0201 and DRB1*03 have been found to be protective and lead to better outcomes, and CCR2, HLA DQ2 and DR3 have been found to be risk factors for worse outcomes [9–12].

7. Differential diagnoses

Many conditions and diseases can cause erythema nodosum, polyarthritis and associated fever. These including: infections, drug reactions, malignancies, inflammatory bowel disease and other rheumatologic conditions. While chest radiograph with findings of hilar adenopathy can significantly increase specificity for Löfgren's syndrome, it is not always necessary and a detailed history and physical should be able to differentiate many of the other differential diagnoses listed below.

7.1 Infections

A wide variety of infections can cause erythema nodosum and arthritis, which can manifest as reactive arthritis or infectious arthritis. These include bacterial: streptococcous, chalymdia, yersinina, salmonella, campylobacter and tubcerculosis. Fungal: coccidiomycosis, histoplasmosis, blastomycosis. Viral: hepatitis B and infectious mononucleosis. Reactive and infectious arthritis generally present initially in the knee joint, which can overlap with Löfgren's syndrome, and the arthritis are also usually self-limited and acute. Therefore it can be difficult to distinguish between the two without chest radiography, but presence of hilar lymphadenopathy should exclude most of the infections listed above. The exception to this is tuberculosis, which can also present with hilar adenopathy, thus it is necessary to obtain tuberculosis skin or interferon-gamma testing to rule out tuberculosis infection.

7.2 Drug reactions

Drug reactions that can cause erythema nodosum include: oral contraceptives, penicillins, sulfonamides, bromides, iodides and TNF Alpha inhibitors. Though drug reactions can cause fever, very rarely do they cause arthritis. Cessation of offending drug also often resolves symptoms. Thus, if there is no presence of acute polyarthritis, distinguishing a drug reaction from Löfgren's syndrome is clear.

7.3 Malignancies

Malignancies that can cause erythema nodosum include lymphoma, leukemia and carcinomas. These malignancies can also be associated with fever, but also very rarely cause arthritis. They can, however, cause hilar lymphadenopathy, thus it is important to delineate presence of acute polyarthritis.

7.4 Inflammatory bowel disease (IBD)

Ulcerative colitis and Crohns disease can cause erythema nodosum with associated fever as well as enteropathic arthritis. Enteropathic arthritis can present sporadically and intermittently, and can be mistaken for acute polyarthritis. Therefore, it is difficult to distinguish between inflammatory bowel disease and Löfgren's syndrome, chest radiography should be obtained to detect for presence of hilar adenopathy. IBD generally does not cause hilar lymphadenopathy.

7.5 Other rheumatologic conditions

Rheumatologic conditions such as Behcet disease and Sweet syndrome can also cause erythema nodosum, arthritis with associated fevers. Behcet syndrome causes polyarthritis of lower extremity joints, very similar to Löfgren's syndrome. Sweet syndrome itself does not cause arthritis, but is associated with rheumatoid arthritis, IBD and Behcet syndrome, all of which can cause arthritis. Sweet syndrome is associated with a characteristic rash that present as erythematous plaques, which should be differentiated from erythema nodosum. Neither condition is associated with hilar lymphadenopathy, thus chest radiography should be obtained to distinguish them from Löfgren's syndrome.

8. Treatment/management

Löfgren's syndrome is largely a self-limited disease, the erythema nodosum, acute polyarthritis and hilar lymphadenopathy resolves usually within a few weeks to months, most cases resolve within 1 year. Polyarthritis has been known to last up to 2 years. Treatment is largely supportive and goal is symptomatic control. NSAIDs are first line for anti-inflammatory properties to ameliorate discomfort of fever, erythema nodosum and arthritis; colchcine can also be used for this purpose. In severe or refractory cases, glucocorticoids can be used, which needs to be tapered off of once symptoms have been resolved. Further interventions with methotrexate or hydroxychloroquine can also be used, and infiximab beyond that [36].

9. Prognosis

Prognosis of Löfgren's syndrome is excellent; most patients achieve complete resolution of symptoms without recurrence in 6 months to 2 years. Cases have been described of recurrence of symptoms or progression to chronic disease, but these are exceedingly rare [35].

10. Conclusions

Löfgren's syndrome is a rare disease that is often misdiagnosed or under diagnosed. The constellation of symptoms of erythema nodosum, acute polyarthritis (most commonly bilaterally in ankle and under 2 months since time of onset) as well as hilar lymphadenopathy in a young patient (under 40 years of age) should raise very high suspicions for this disease. Prompt recognition and treatment of this disease can save much stress and pain for patients afflicted by it.

Conflict of interest

The authors declare no conflict of interest.

Author details

Shiyu Wang[1*] and Shailendra Singh[2]

1 White River Health System, Batesville, AR, USA

2 Unity Healthy System, Searcy, AR, USA

*Address all correspondence to: shiyuwang0@gmail.com

References

[1] Thomas KW, Hunninghake GW. Sarcoidosis. JAMA. 2003 Jun 25;289(24):3300-3303. doi: 10.1001/jama.289.24.3300. PMID: 12824213.

[2] Newman LS, Rose CS, Maier LA. Sarcoidosis. N Engl J Med. 1997 Apr 24;336(17):1224-34. doi: 10.1056/NEJM199704243361706. Erratum in: N Engl J Med 1997 Jul 10;337(2):139. PMID: 9110911.

[3] Arkema EV, Cozier YC. Epidemiology of sarcoidosis: current findings and future directions. *Ther Adv Chronic Dis*. 2018;9(11):227-240. Published 2018 Aug 24. doi:10.1177/2040622318790197

[4] Rybicki BA, Major M, Popovich J Jr, Maliarik MJ, Iannuzzi MC. Racial differences in sarcoidosis incidence: a 5-year study in a health maintenance organization. Am J Epidemiol. 1997 Feb 1;145(3):234-241. doi: 10.1093/oxfordjournals.aje.a009096. PMID: 9012596.

[5] Baughman RP, Lower EE, du Bois RM. Sarcoidosis. Lancet. 2003 Mar 29;361(9363):1111-1118. doi: 10.1016/S0140-6736(03)12888-7. PMID: 12672326.

[6] Visser H, Vos K, Zanelli E, Verduyn W, Schreuder GM, Speyer I, Breedveld FC, Hazes JM. Sarcoid arthritis: clinical characteristics, diagnostic aspects, and risk factors. Ann Rheum Dis. 2002 Jun;61(6):499-504. doi: 10.1136/ard.61.6.499. PMID: 12006321; PMCID: PMC1754119.

[7] Rubio-Rivas M, Franco J, Corbella X. Sarcoidosis presenting with and without Löfgren's syndrome: Clinical, radiological and behavioral differences observed in a group of 691patients. Joint Bone Spine. 2020 Mar;87(2):141-147. doi: 10.1016/j.jbspin.2019.10.001. Epub 2019 Oct 11. PMID: 31606494.

[8] Grunewald J, Eklund A. Sex-specific manifestations of Löfgren's syndrome. Am J Respir Crit Care Med. 2007;175(1):40-44. doi:10.1164/rccm.200608-1197OC

[9] Sato H, Grutters JC, Pantelidis P, Mizzon AN, Ahmad T, Van Houte AJ, Lammers JW, Van Den Bosch JM, Welsh KI, Du Bois RM. HLA-DQB1*0201: a marker for good prognosis in British and Dutch patients with sarcoidosis. Am J Respir Cell Mol Biol. 2002 Oct;27(4):406-412. doi: 10.1165/rcmb.4782. PMID: 12356573.

[10] Grunewald J, Eklund A. Löfgren's syndrome: human leukocyte antigen strongly influences the disease course. Am J Respir Crit Care Med. 2009 Feb 15;179(4):307-312. doi: 10.1164/rccm.200807-1082OC. Epub 2008 Nov 7. PMID: 18996998.

[11] Spagnolo P, Renzoni EA, Wells AU, Sato H, Grutters JC, Sestini P, Abdallah A, Gramiccioni E, Ruven HJ, du Bois RM, Welsh KI. C-C chemokine receptor 2 and sarcoidosis: association with Lofgren's syndrome. Am J Respir Crit Care Med. 2003 Nov 15;168(10):1162-1166. doi: 10.1164/rccm.200303-456OC. Epub 2003 Jul 25. PMID: 12882757.

[12] Kremer JM. Histologic findings in siblings with acute sarcoid arthritis: association with the B8,DR3 phenotype. J Rheumatol. 1986 Jun;13(3):593-597. PMID: 3488404.

[13] Rybicki BA, Iannuzzi MC, Frederick MM, Thompson BW, Rossman MD, Bresnitz EA, Terrin ML, Moller DR, Barnard J, Baughman RP, DePalo L, Hunninghake G, Johns C, Judson MA, Knatterud GL, McLennan G, Newman LS, Rabin DL, Rose C, Teirstein AS, Weinberger SE, Yeager H, Cherniack R; ACCESS Research Group. Familial aggregation of sarcoidosis. A case-control etiologic study of sarcoidosis (ACCESS). Am J Respir Crit Care Med. 2001 Dec

1;164(11):2085-2091. doi: 10.1164/ajrccm.164.11.2106001. PMID: 11739139.

[14] Balmes JR, Abraham JL, Dweik RA, Fireman E, Fontenot AP, Maier LA, Muller-Quernheim J, Ostiguy G, Pepper LD, Saltini C, Schuler CR, Takaro TK, Wambach PF; ATS Ad Hoc Committee on Beryllium Sensitivity and Chronic Beryllium Disease. An official American Thoracic Society statement: diagnosis and management of beryllium sensitivity and chronic beryllium disease. Am J Respir Crit Care Med. 2014 Nov 15;190(10):e34-e59. doi: 10.1164/rccm.201409-1722ST. PMID: 25398119.

[15] Werfel U, Schneider J, Rödelsperger K, Kotter J, Popp W, Woitowitz HJ, Zieger G. Sarcoid granulomatosis after zirconium exposure with multiple organ involvement. Eur Respir J. 1998 Sep;12(3):750. doi: 10.1183/09031936.98.12030750. PMID: 9762810.

[16] Cai HR, Cao M, Meng FQ, Wei JY. Pulmonary sarcoid-like granulomatosis induced by aluminum dust: report of a case and literature review. Chin Med J (Engl). 2007 Sep 5;120(17):1556-1560. PMID: 17908469.

[17] Izbicki G, Chavko R, Banauch GI, Weiden MD, Berger KI, Aldrich TK, Hall C, Kelly KJ, Prezant DJ. World Trade Center "sarcoid-like" granulomatous pulmonary disease in New York City Fire Department rescue workers. Chest. 2007 May;131(5):1414-1423. doi: 10.1378/chest.06-2114. Epub 2007 Mar 30. PMID: 17400664.

[18] Ferrara G, Valentini D, Rao M, Wahlström J, Grunewald J, Larsson LO, Brighenti S, Dodoo E, Zumla A, Maeurer M. Humoral immune profiling of mycobacterial antigen recognition in sarcoidosis and Löfgren's syndrome using high-content peptide microarrays. Int J Infect Dis. 2017 Mar;56:167-175. doi: 10.1016/j.ijid.2017.01.021. Epub 2017 Jan 31. PMID: 28159576.

[19] Ishige I, Eishi Y, Takemura T, Kobayashi I, Nakata K, Tanaka I, Nagaoka S, Iwai K, Watanabe K, Takizawa T, Koike M. Propionibacterium acnes is the most common bacterium commensal in peripheral lung tissue and mediastinal lymph nodes from subjects without sarcoidosis. Sarcoidosis Vasc Diffuse Lung Dis. 2005 Mar;22(1):33-42. PMID: 15881278.

[20] Saboor SA, Johnson NM, McFadden J. Detection of mycobacterial DNA in sarcoidosis and tuberculosis with polymerase chain reaction. Lancet. 1992 Apr 25;339(8800):1012-1015. doi: 10.1016/0140-6736(92)90535-b. PMID: 1349051.

[21] Burke WM, Keogh A, Maloney PJ, Delprado W, Bryant DH, Spratt P. Transmission of sarcoidosis via cardiac transplantation. Lancet. 1990 Dec 22-29;336(8730):1579. doi: 10.1016/0140-6736(90)93354-r. PMID: 1979389.

[22] Bhagat R, Rizzieri DA, Vredenburgh JJ, Chao NJ, Folz RJ. Pulmonary sarcoidosis following stem cell transplantation: is it more than a chance occurrence? Chest. 2004 Aug;126(2):642-644. doi: 10.1378/chest.126.2.642. PMID: 15302757.

[23] Ionescu DN, Hunt JL, Lomago D, Yousem SA. Recurrent sarcoidosis in lung transplant allografts: granulomas are of recipient origin. Diagn Mol Pathol. 2005 Sep;14(3):140-145. doi: 10.1097/01.pas.0000176765.26047.6f. PMID: 16106194.

[24] Sakthivel P, Bruder D. Mechanism of granuloma formation in sarcoidosis. Curr Opin Hematol. 2017 Jan;24(1):59-65. doi: 10.1097/MOH.0000000000000301. PMID: 27755127.

[25] Broos CE, Hendriks RW, Kool M. T-cell immunology in sarcoidosis: Disruption of a delicate balance between helper and regulatory T-cells. Curr Opin Pulm Med. 2016 Sep;22(5):476-483. doi:

10.1097/MCP.0000000000000303. PMID: 27379969.

[26] Judson MA. The Clinical Features of Sarcoidosis: A Comprehensive Review. Clin Rev Allergy Immunol. 2015 Aug;49(1):63-78. doi: 10.1007/s12016-014-8450-y. PMID: 25274450.

[27] Kunz M, Beutel S, Bröcker E. Leucocyte activation in erythema nodosum. Clin Exp Dermatol. 1999 Sep;24(5):396-401. doi: 10.1046/j.1365-2230.1999.00511.x. PMID: 10564331.

[28] Ponhold W. Das Löfgren-Syndrom: Die akute Form der Sarkoidose [The Löfgren syndrome: acute sarcoidosis (author's transl)]. Rontgenblatter. 1977 Jun;30(6):325-7. German. PMID: 897518.

[29] Roberto J. Barrios, Chapter 17 - Other Interstitial Lung Diseases, Editor(s): Dani S. Zander, Carol F. Farver, In The Foundations in Diagnostic Pathology Series, Pulmonary Pathology, Churchill Livingstone, 2008, Pages 348-373, ISBN 9780443067419, https://doi.org/10.1016/B978-0-443-06741-9.50023-9.

[30] Visser H, Vos K, Zanelli E, et al. Sarcoid arthritis: clinical characteristics, diagnostic aspects, and risk factors. Ann Rheum Dis. 2002;61(6):499-504. doi:10.1136/ard.61.6.499

[31] Johard U, Eklund A. Recurrent Löfgren's syndrome in three patients with sarcoidosis. Sarcoidosis. 1993 Sep;10(2):125-127. PMID: 8140298.

[32] MAYOCK RL, BERTRAND P, MORRISON CE, SCOTT JH. MANIFESTATIONS OF SARCOIDOSIS. ANALYSIS OF 145 PATIENTS, WITH A REVIEW OF NINE SERIES SELECTED FROM THE LITERATURE. Am J Med. 1963 Jul;35:67-89. doi: 10.1016/0002-9343(63)90165-7. PMID: 14046006.

[33] Koyama T, Ueda H, Togashi K, Umeoka S, Kataoka M, Nagai S. Radiologic manifestations of sarcoidosis in various organs. Radiographics. 2004 Jan-Feb;24(1):87-104. doi: 10.1148/rg.241035076. PMID: 14730039.

[34] Winterbauer RH, Lammert J, Selland M, Wu R, Corley D, Springmeyer SC. Bronchoalveolar lavage cell populations in the diagnosis of sarcoidosis. Chest. 1993 Aug;104(2):352-361. doi: 10.1378/chest.104.2.352. PMID: 8339618.

[35] Sejdic A, Graudal N, Baslund B. Clinical and biochemical presentation of sarcoidosis with high and normal serum angiotensin-converting enzyme. Scand J Rheumatol. 2018 Nov;47(6):487-490. doi: 10.1080/03009742.2017.1420818. Epub 2018 Jun 22. PMID: 29929412.

[36] Zisman DA, Shorr AF, Lynch JP 3rd. Sarcoidosis involving the musculoskeletal system. Semin Respir Crit Care Med. 2002 Dec;23(6):555-570. doi: 10.1055/s-2002-36520. PMID: 16088651.

Section 3

Rare Neoplastic Diseases

Chapter 4

Childhood Langerhans Cell Histiocytosis: Epidemiology, Clinical Presentations, Prognostic Factors, and Therapeutic Approaches

Katharina Sterlich and Milen Minkov

Abstract

Childhood LCH is a rare disease, affecting 4–9 per 1,000,000 children below the age of 15 years. It is driven by somatic mutations in the MAPK pathway, arising in myeloid marrow progenitors. Both genders are affected by a slight male preponderance. The clinical spectrum of LCH varies from a single lesion affecting one organ system to severe multisystem disease with dysfunction of vital organs. Likewise, variable and unpredictable is its course, spanning from self-limiting course to progression with lethal outcome. Recognized unfavorable prognostic factors are the involvement of hematopoiesis, liver, and spleen, as well as non-response to systemic treatment. Recent studies suggest that patients carrying the BRAFV600E mutation may have a more severe clinical phenotype and less favorable prognosis. The combination of prednisolone and vinblastine is the standard first-line treatment for disseminated disease. Second-line options used in clinical practice are not well evidenced. Inhibitors of the MAPK pathway are a promising alternative option.

Keywords: langerhans cell histiocytosis, epidemiology, manifestations, prognostic factors, treatment

1. Introduction

LCH is a rare disease with a variety of presentations and outcomes. Indeed, for most of its history, it was thought to be several different entities until sufficient cases were described that made the spectrum of this disease clearer.

The descriptive approach in medicine in the early 20th century and the extremely heterogeneous clinical presentation of LCH led to the fact that different manifestations of the disease were described as separate syndromes. Thus, the history of the disease began with the description of the Hand-Schüller-Christian syndrome, [1–3], the Letterer-Siwe disease, [4, 5] and the eosinophilic granuloma [6].

In 1953, Dr. L. Lichtenstein in a critical review of the literature introduced a unifying concept, stating that the conditions previously designated eosinophilic

IntechOpen

granuloma of bone, Letterer-Siwe disease and Hand-Schüller-Christian disease, are interrelated manifestations of a single disease [7]. The name "histiocytosis X" was suggested to underscore the unknown origin of the disease.

In 1973, Dr. Christian Nezelof, a French pediatric pathologist, proposed the Langerhans cells as the origin of histiocytosis X [8]. His hypothesis was based on morphologic similarities (e.g. Birbeck granule, a cytoplasmic pentalaminar structure with a tennis racket shape) between normal Langerhans cells and the abnormal cells in histiocytosis X. Since then the disease is referred to as Langerhans cell histiocytosis.

2. Epidemiology

The estimated incidence of LCH is 4–9 children younger than 15 years per million [9–12]. The peak incidence of childhood LCH is between 0 and 4 years [13]. There is a relation between age at manifestation and disease extent, younger children have more disseminated disease [14]. All large epidemiologic studies report a male predominance in the range of 1.2–1.5 [9–12]. The causes and risk factors for developing LCH are unclear [15]. However, the unique patterns of presentation, ranging from localized bone lesions with spontaneous regression to disseminated forms with involvement of multiple organs, suggest a complex pathogenesis. Familial clustering, particularly the observation of increased incidence in monozygotic twins, have suggested the presence of a germline predisposition at least for a proportion of cases [16, 17]. In addition, population-based studies have shown differences in the incidence of disseminated LCH by race and ethnic group; a higher incidence has been reported for Hispanics and a lower incidence for blacks [18]. Studies have also shown a correlation with maternal and neonatal infections, [15, 19, 20] lack of childhood vaccinations, [15, 20] family history of thyroid disease, [15] in vitro fertilization, [21] and feeding problems and transfusions during infancy [19]. Finally, lower socioeconomic conditions have been associated with an increased incidence of disseminated LCH [18].

3. Clinical presentation

The clinical presentations of LCH range from incidentally detected asymptomatic bone lesions to severe multisystem disease manifesting with disseminated rash, fever, failure to thrive, enlarged liver and spleen and transfusion-dependent cytopenia (**Figure 1**). The disease can present with insidious nonspecific manifestations such as fever, impaired appetite, anxiety, and sleep disturbances, particularly in infants. Virtually all organ systems can be affected either individually (single system LCH; SS-LCH) or in different combinations (multisystem LCH; MS-LCH). Hence, LCH can mimic a large spectrum of diseases (**Table 1**). Frequent, though unspecific manifestations are: bone pain, soft tissue swelling ("bumps") in the head and neck area, persistent polymorphic skin eruptions, mucous membrane ulcerations, respiratory symptoms (cough, shortness of breath, chest pain), enlargement of the liver, spleen and lymph nodes, growth failure, polyuria with polydipsia or, rarely, neurological symptoms.

The organs mostly affected are bone (80%), skin (33%) and pituitary (25%). The hematopoietic system, spleen, liver and lungs are affected in up to 15%, lymph nodes in 5–10% and the central nervous system without the pituitary in 2–4% of the patients [22].

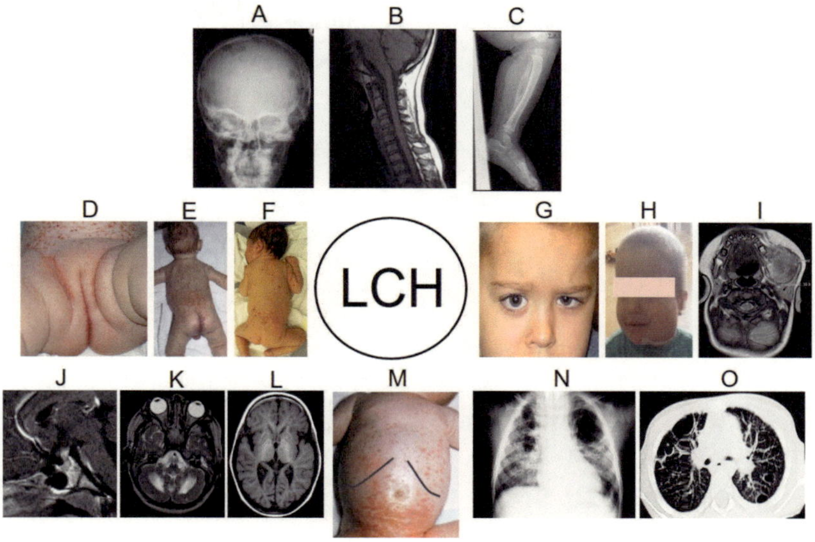

Figure 1.
Spectrum of clinical manifestations. Bone lesions in the skull (A) with irregular punched out appearance, vertebra (B) with partial collapse of the vertebral body, and the tibia (C) with periosteal reaction and bone deformity; Cutaneous manifestations: purpuric rash with erythema and maceration of the inguinal folds resembling diaper dermatitis (D), characteristic confluent maculopapular rash with purpuric appearance and crusting on the trunk (E), and papulonodular reddish-brown rash in a newborn (F); Right-sided proptosis caused by a lesion of the orbital bones (G); Jawbone lesion presenting as a massive soft-tissue swelling (H) and the respective MRI findings (I); J - Thickening of the pituitary infundibulum, manifesting as central diabetes insipidus; Characteristic non-granulomatous lesions of the cerebellum (K) and the basal ganglia (L); Massive hepatosplenomegaly and skin rash in severe multisystem LCH (M); Pulmonary LCH with bullae visible on radiography (N) and combination of nodules and cysts on CT scan (O).

3.1 Skeleton

Flat bones and particularly the cranial bones are most commonly affected. Other common locations in decreasing order are the long bones of the extremities, the vertebral bodies and the pelvic bones. The proximal bones of the extremities are more frequently involved than the distal ones. The bones of the hands and feet are usually sparred. The lesions are characteristically located in the diaphysis or metaphysis, but the epiphysis can be affected as well.

Vertebral lesions typically localize in the vertebral body, vertebral arch, transverse or spinous process and present with pain, kyphoscoliosis, or neurological deficits due to compression of the spinal cord [23]. While vertebra plana in LCH are rare, LCH is the leading cause of vertebra plana in children.

Unilateral or bilateral lesions in the temporal bone range from unspecific opacification of the mastoid cells with minimal bone destruction, to extensive osseous destruction and intracranial soft tissue infiltration. The most common symptoms are recurrent or persistent otitis, mucopurulent otorrhea, swelling of the mastoid, and eczema or polyps of the ear canal. In rare cases of inner ear involvement, hearing loss, dizziness or paralysis of the facial nerve also occur.

Lesions of the orbital bones in LCH are mostly unilateral and have exclusively extraconal location, typically affecting the roof and the lateral wall [24]. They manifest with lid swelling (with or without inflammatory appearance), palpable mass, or proptosis. The differentials of orbital involvement include acute infections, inflammatory pseudotumor, hemangioma, rhabdomyosarcoma, retinoblastoma, metastatic neuroblastoma, lymphoma, and optic glioma. However, other histiocytic disorders, such as juvenile xanthogranuloma, Erdheim-Chester disease, and Rosai-Dorfman disease can present with orbital involvement as well.

Affected organ	Manifestation/finding	Differentials
Skin	Vesicles and bullae (most common in early infancy)	Erythema toxicum Herpes simplex Varicella
	Dermatitis (most frequently scalp, diaper area, or axilla) Nodules ("blueberry muffin" like) Petechia Pruritic rash	Seborrheic dermatitis Mastocytosis Juvenile xanthogranuloma Neuroblastoma Infant leukemia Intrauterine infections Scabies
Bone	Vertebral lesions (vertebra plana)	Chronic relapsing multifocal osteomyelitis (CRMO) Leukemia/Lymphoma Aneurysmal bone cyst Erdheim-Chester disease Ewing sarcoma Osteosarcoma Metabolic bone diseases
	Temporal bone	Chronic otitis media Mastoiditis Cholesteatoma Soft tissue sarcoma
	Orbit	Acute infection (preseptal cellulitis) Dermoid cyst Erdheim–Chester disease Pseudoinflammatory tumor Rhabdomyosarcoma Neuroblastoma
	Lytic lesions of the long bones	Septic osteomyelitis CRMO Aneurysmal bone cyst Bone angiomatosis (Gorham disease) Fibrous dysplasia Giant cell tumor of bone Atypical mycobacterial infection Osteogenic sarcoma Ewing's sarcoma
Lung	Respiratory symptoms, reticular lesions (nodules and cysts)	Mycobacterial or other pulmonary infections Sarcoidosis
Liver	Hepatomegaly, jaundice with direct hyperbilirubinemia Hypoalbuminemia	Chronic destructive cholangitis Metabolic diseases Hepatitis Diseases obstructing biliary tract Inherited diseases of bilirubin conjugation Toxic (Reye syndrome) Neonatal hemochromatosis Chronic inflammatory bowel disease
Endocrine glands (pituitary, thyroid)	Polyuria/polydipsia, growth failure, hypothyroidism, hypogonadism	Renal diabetes insipidus Head trauma Germ cell tumors of CNS Lymphatic hypophysitis Non-LCH histiocytoses

Table 1.
Common differential diagnoses of LCH.

Jaw involvement can present with gingival hyperplasia or ulceration, extensive dissolution of the jawbone structure with tooth loosening ("floating teeth") or loss.

3.2 Skin

Skin is the second most frequently involved organ system after the skeleton overall. In patients younger than two years, it is even the most frequently involved organ. Cutaneous involvement is typically representative of multisystem disease, as 87–93% also have systemic involvement. Cutaneous lesions may be either circumscribed (nodular) or spread and confluent (rash).

They typically present as pinpoint erythematous or skin-colored papules or pustules. The morphology can mimic a seborrheic dermatitis-like or an eczematous erythematous, skin-colored, or brown petechial rash with or without scale, scabbing, crusting, and/or purpura. In infants, a seborrheic dermatitis-like rash on the scalp often causes LCH to be misdiagnosed as seborrheic dermatitis, while groin involvement can mimic treatment-resistant, recurring diaper dermatitis [25].

Nail involvement is rare, but can present as subungual pustules, hemorrhage, or hyperkeratosis, purpuric striae, purulent discharge, longitudinal grooving, onycholysis, paronychia, and pitting [25].

3.3 Lymph nodes

Enlarged lymph nodes are rarely the only manifestation of a single system LCH. The lymphadenopathy encountered in the setting of multisystem disease is usually mild to moderate.

3.4 Bone marrow

Peripheral blood cytopenia in LCH patients, often referred to as "hematologic dysfunction", is a sign of severe disease and heralds unfavorable prognosis. For decades, the terms "hematopoietic dysfunction" and "bone marrow involvement" were interchangeably used in the literature [26]. Bone marrow studies in LCH patients using immunochemical staining for CD1a or molecular markers (BRAFV600E), have found increased proportion of histiocytes compared to controls, but their numbers did not correlate well with disease extent and severity [26, 27]. Strikingly, the phagocytosis in the bone marrow, which better correlates to disease severity, is carried out by CD1a-negative macrophages. Although the exact mechanisms leading to peripheral cytopenia remain uncovered, it is clear that it is not due to marrow infiltration in most cases, and is probably due to increased phagocytosis or inflammatory marrow suppression.

3.5 Spleen

Enlargement of the spleen in LCH occurs exclusively in the setting of MS-LCH. It occurs in 15–30% of the patients mostly coinciding with hematopoietic and liver involvement.

3.6 Liver

Liver involvement occurs exclusively in children with MS-LCH. Patients may present with hepatomegaly only or with functional impairment (elevated liver enzymes, hypoproteinemia and hypoalbuminemia) and/or jaundice.

Two patterns of liver dysfunction can been seen in children: one with predominant hypoproteinemia/hypoalbuminemia ± mild elevation of transaminases and bilirubin; and a less common cholestatic one, due to progressive sclerosing cholangitis [28]. The former is usually combined with prominent constitutional symptoms, and is characteristically observed in the setting of active LCH, while the latter is usually seen as a disease consequence and often without concomitant activity of LCH elsewhere.

3.7 Lungs

Isolated pulmonary LCH (also known as primary pulmonary LCH) is extremely rare in children, accounting for less than 1% of all pediatric LCH cases. However, pulmonary involvement in the setting of MS-LCH presents at diagnosis in about 25% of cases [29]. The most common clinical symptoms are tachypnea, cyanosis, chest pain and chronic or persistent cough. Characteristic imaging findings are symmetric bilateral reticulo-nodular opacities ± bullae on radiography and combination of nodules and cysts on CT. Histopathological verification of lung involvement in children with confirmed LCH is required only in case of uncharacteristic or inconsistent imaging findings. Symptom severity and time course can vary. In rare cases, excessive tissue destruction and cyst formation can result in (recurring) life-threatening pneumothorax. Honeycombing with end-stage lung disease is a rare permanent sequela of pediatric LCH.

3.8 Gastrointestinal tract

Gastrointestinal involvement in LCH (GI-LCH) is infrequent, accounting for about 2–3% of the pediatric series. It usually occurs in the setting of a multisystem LCH, and depending of the affected gut segment, clinically presents with vomiting, abdominal pain, protein-losing enteropathy, bloody and non-bloody diarrhea, malabsorption, and failure to thrive. The prognostic value of gut involvement remains controversial but currently published paper suggests unfavorable impact on survival [30].

3.9 Endocrine system

Involvement of the hypothalamic–pituitary axis and the resulting central diabetes insipidus (CDI) and dysfunction of the anterior pituitary are a hallmark of LCH. Characteristic findings on MRI are hypothalamic mass, infundibular thickening, and lacking posterior bright spot. CDI manifests with polyuria and polydipsia, and can be the inaugural manifestation of LCH or develop later during disease course. Its prevalence in children with multisystem LCH is between 20 and 35%. Loss of the hormones of the anterior pituitary is less common than CDI. In order of decreasing frequency, pituitary LCH can cause growth hormone (growth failure), thyroid-stimulating hormone (hypothyroidism), adrenocorticotropic hormone (hypocortisolism), luteinizing and follicle-stimulating hormone (hypogonadism) loss. Thyroid involvement is rare, with only 75 cases reported in the literature [25]. It can manifest with gland enlargement due to diffuse or nodular lesions, but the function is mostly preserved.

3.10 Thymus

Thymus involvement is a rare event with estimated frequency of 1–2% and mostly seen in young children with MS-LCH [31]. Typical imaging findings are enlargement of the gland, cysts and calcifications. Sonography allows for a reliable non-invasive evaluation of the thymus [31].

3.11 Central nervous system (CNS-LCH)

LCH can affect brain in different ways and result in a variety of manifestations and clinical problems. With respect to risk factors, clinical presentation, imaging findings and the classification of CNS-LCH, the interested readers are referred to two dedicated review papers [32, 33]. For the purposes of clinical management LCH of the brain is divided into granulomatous (tumorous) and non-granulomatous (neurodegenerative) CNS-LCH.

Granulomatous (tumorous) lesions of the CNS are defined as space-occupying lesions involving brain structures. Any of the following brain regions may be involved either by isolated lesions or in the context of multisystem disease: hypothalamic–pituitary region (HPR), pineal gland, meninges or choroid plexus [32, 33].

Non-granulomatous (neurodegenerative) lesions encompass two subtypes [32, 33]:

- Radiological neurodegeneration or LCH-associated abnormal CNS imaging (LACI). This term refers to typical signal changes on two consecutive MRI scans performed within an interval of at least 3 months without related clinical manifestations.

- Clinical neurodegeneration or LCH-associated abnormal CNS symptoms (LACS). This clinical syndrome is defined as the presence of overt neurological or neuropsychological deficits in the context of consistent radiological findings.

4. Prognostic factors

The broad spectrum of clinical manifestations and the variability of disease course and outcome makes prediction of prognosis quite challenging. Attempts to split the disease into categories with distinct prognosis led to elaboration of a number of staging and scoring systems [34–37]. Established prognostic factors in pediatric LCH are disease extent (SS-LCH vs. MC-LCH), involvement of organs crucial for survival (risk organs, e.g. hematopoiesis, liver, spleen) and early response to systemic treatment [38].

SS-LCH has an excellent prognosis, with a survival rate of nearly 100% and a 5-year recurrence rate of less than 20% [39]. Relapses are usually limited to skeleton and posterior pituitary (diabetes insipidus) and therefore do not affect survival [39, 40].

MS-LCH is a broad category encompassing patients with involvement of two to more than seven organ systems. In 1975, E. Lahey introduced the definition of organ dysfunction [41]. Lahey's definition has been in use for treatment stratification for many decades, and in the 1990s, it was replaced by the definition of "risk organ involvement" [34, 35, 37, 42].

Response to an initial 6-week course of systemic therapy has proved to be an additional independent prognostic factor [37, 43–45]. Risk organ involvement at diagnosis and lack of response to 6-weeks of systemic treatment define a subgroup of MS-LCH patients with survival of only 20–40% [46].

The French LCH Working Group has developed a disease activity score, which is suitable, for longitudinal objective assessment of disease burden and treatment success [47].

5. Pretreatment patient evaluation and stratification

The experience from institutional cohorts, registries and clinical trials has unequivocally proven that treatment of LCH has to be tailored to disease extent and severity and to take into account mortality risk. For this purpose, standardized clinical evaluation of each patient at initial diagnosis and relapse is mandatory [22, 48, 49]. The mandatory set of laboratory tests and imaging is presented in **Table 2**. Further investigations to be performed upon specific indications are listed in **Table 3**. Based on the results of the initial evaluation the patients are attributed to one of the disease extent categories of the clinical classification of LCH (**Table 4**). The empirical clinical classification of LCH was developed for the purposes of treatment stratification. The definitions of risk organ involvement are summarized in **Table 5**.

Test	Description
Blood counts	• Hemoglobin • White blood cell and differential count • Platelet count
Erythrocyte sedimentation rate	
Blood chemistry	• Total protein, albumin, bilirubin, ALT (SGPT), AST (SGOT), alkaline phosphatase, γGT • BUN, creatinine, electrolytes • Ferritin
Coagulation studies	• PT, APTT/PTT, fibrinogen
Urinalysis	• Specific gravity and osmolality in an early morning urine sample
Imaging:	
Abdominal ultrasound	Size and structure of liver and spleen?
Chest radiography	Reticulo-nodular opacifications, bullae?
Skeletal survey (radiography, PET/CT, whole-body MRI*)	* Marrow signal alterations detected by MRI need confirmation. Only bone lesions confirmed by x-ray, CT, PET/CT, or biopsy count for stratification.

Table 2.
Mandatory baseline evaluation upon initial diagnosis, progression or relapse.

Indication	Test
Risk organ involvement	• HLA typing
Bi- or pancytopenia, or persistent unexplained single cytopenia	• Bone marrow aspirate & trephine biopsy to also exclude causes other than LCH
Liver dysfunction	• Liver biopsy only recommended if there is clinically significant liver involvement and the result will alter treatment i.e. to differentiate active LCH from sclerosing cholangitis
Lung involvement (abnormal radiography or symptoms/signs suggestive for lung involvement)	• Low dose multi-detector volume-CT is preferable to high-resolution CT of the lungs • Lung function test (if age appropriate)
Abnormal lung CT AND findings not characteristic for LCH or suspicion for atypical infection*	• Bronchoalveolar lavage (BAL), >5% CD1a-positive cells in BAL fluid is diagnostic in non-smokers • Lung biopsy (if BAL not diagnostic)
Suspected craniofacial bone lesions including maxilla (mandible excluded)	• MRI of head • CT could be considered in addition, if needed for better view of skeletal lesions
Suspected vertebral lesions	• MRI of spine (to exclude spinal cord compression and evaluate soft tissue masses)
Visual or neurological abnormalities	• MRI of head • Neurology assessment • Neuropsychometric assessment
Suspected endocrine abnormality (i.e. short stature, growth failure, polyuria, polydipsia, hypothalamic syndromes, precocious or delayed puberty) and/or imaging abnormality of hypothalamus/ pituitary	• Endocrine assessment (including water deprivation test and dynamic tests of the anterior pituitary) • MRI of brain (focussed on hypothalamic–pituitary region)

Indication	Test
Aural discharge or suspected hearing impairment/mastoid involvement	• Formal hearing assessment • MRI of head • CT of temporal bone
Unexplained chronic diarrhea, failure to thrive or evidence of malabsorption	• Endoscopy and biopsy

In case of verified LCH in other organs, biopsy is indicated ONLY if the pulmonary findings on CT are inconsistent with LCH or atypical infection is suspected.

Table 3.
Laboratory investigations and imaging recommended upon specific indications.

Disease category	Definition
Single system LCH (SS-LCH)	One organ/system involved (uni- or multifocal): • Bone unifocal (single bone) or multifocal (>1 bone) • Skin • Lymph node (not the draining lymph node of another LCH lesion) • Lungs • Central nervous system • Other (e.g. thyroid, thymus)
Multisystem LCH (MS-LCH)	Two or more organs/systems involved: • Without risk organ involvement • With risk organ involvement (at least one of the following: hematopoietic system, liver, or spleen)

Table 4.
Clinical classification of LCH.

Risk organ	Involvement criteria
Hematopoiesis (with or without bone marrow infiltration*)	At least 2 of the following: • Anemia: hemoglobin <100 g/L (<10 g/dl), infants <90 g/L (<9.0 g/dl), not due to other causes e.g. iron deficiency • Leukocytopenia: leukocytes <4,0 x109/l (4,000/μL) • Thrombocytopenia: platelets <100 x109/l (100.000/μL)
Spleen	• Enlargement >2 cm below costal margin in the midclavicular line**
Liver	• Enlargement >3 cm below costal margin in the midclavicular line** • and/or • dysfunction (i.e. hypoproteinemia <55 g/L, hypoalbuminemia <25 g/L, not due to other causes • and/or • histopathological findings of active disease

**Bone marrow infiltration is defined as presence of CD1a positive cells on marrow slides. The clinical significance of marrow CD1a positivity is still unclear. In cases of severe progressive disease, prominent hemophagocytosis, as well as hypocellularity, myelodysplasia or myelofibrosis may be found.*
***Enlargement in cm below the costal margin as assessed by palpation or sonography.*

Table 5.
Definition of risk organ involvement.

6. Treatment

Patients with single skeletal lesions usually do not need systemic treatment, except for large symptomatic lesions or lesions in weight-bearing bones, which are not easily accessible for surgical treatment. Treatment of isolated cutaneous LCH is controversial, but if topical treatments fail, systemic treatment needs consideration in infants.

Multifocal skeletal disease and MS-LCH indicate systemic treatment.

6.1 Approach to localized (single-system single site) LCH

Randomized prospective trials for the treatment of localized LCH are not available. Therefore, current treatment recommendations for localized LCH based on experience gained from retrospective cohorts and non-randomized controlled trials [39, 50].

According to existing clinical experience, the majority of patients with localized LCH (mostly confined to skeleton) do not need systemic treatment. Established treatment options range from expectant attitude, through surgery or topical drug application, to systemic therapy in selected cases. Decisive for the treatment choice in unifocal skeletal LCH is the location (weight-bearing bones or imminent compression of adjacent structures), the size, the surgical accessibility, the presence of considerable adjacent soft-tissue mass, pain or functional impairment, and the risk of permanent consequences.

A best practice based treatment approach to SS-LCH is depicted on **Figure 2**.

6.1.1 Wait and watch

A "wait and see" approach is justified in small asymptomatic osseous or cutaneous lesions in view of the high likelihood for spontaneous healing.

6.1.2 Surgery

Surgical procedures such as biopsy, curettage, or resection are used to treat solitary bone lesions, solitary affected lymph nodes, or solitary circumscribed nodular skin lesions. A biopsy is necessary to confirm the diagnosis and at the same time represents a healing stimulus. Clinical experience showed that radical surgery is not necessary and usually not useful in localized LCH [22, 51]. Wide surgical resection

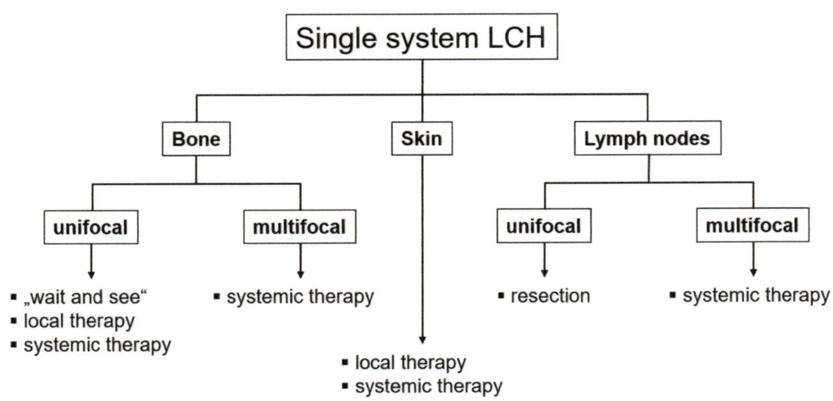

Figure 2.
Treatment approach to single system LCH.

is particularly harmful in skull vault, jawbone lesions, as it impedes bone remodeling, and causes permanent defects, which are unlikely in non-resected lesions.

6.1.3 Topical steroids

An intralesional application of crystalline methylprednisolone (100-150 mg) in symptomatic bone lesion can quickly bring about a reduction in symptoms and facilitated cure [52, 53].

6.1.4 Radiation therapy

Because of its potential to induce secondary malignancies, radiotherapy at a low dose (6–10 Gy) is nowadays limited to specific indications (for example, imminent compression of vital structures (e.g. the spinal cord or the optic nerve).

6.1.5 Systemic therapy

In case of large, symptomatic lesions, which are not easily accessible and bear high likelihood for pathologic fractures and permanent consequences, mild systemic treatment of short duration (3–6 months) using the same regimen as in disseminated LCH, may be the preferable option for local disease control.

6.2 Treatment of disseminated (multifocal skeletal and multisystem) LCH

Multifocal skeletal and multisystem LCH (earlier unified under the term disseminated LCH) have been traditionally considered an indication for systemic treatment. While there is a general agreement on the indication of systemic therapy for patients with MS-LCH, the value of systemic therapy for multifocal skeletal SS-LCH is less well documented and still needs evaluation in controlled prospective trials [46, 50, 54, 55]. A number of individual drugs, drug combinations and regimens have been tested in LCH since the 1960s. Most trials before the era of international cooperation have pooled patients with varying clinical presentation, course, and prognosis to gain meaningful numbers [56]. Methodological weaknesses and inappropriate sample size lead to contradicting results, and most of the early trials are of historic importance only.

The current standard of care foots on evidence of the consecutive clinical trials of the Histiocyte Society [42, 44, 57]. The cumulative evidence of the empirical trials LCH I-III can be summarized as follows:

- The standard front-line therapy for patients with MS-LCH treated outside of controlled clinical trials should consist of a 6–12 weeks of initial therapy (oral steroids and weekly vinblastine injections), followed by pulses of prednisolone/vinblastine every 3 weeks, for a total treatment duration of 12 months.

- Patients with risk organ involvement (particularly those with bi-, pancytopenia and liver dysfunction), who do not respond to 6 weeks of standard treatment have particularly dismal prognosis (survival less than 50%). This small subgroup categorized as "very high risk" deserves treatment intensification. To date only few options have shown promising results in the treatment of severe progressive LCH in small series and pilot trials [58–63]. Their applicability is limited by either high toxicity (cladribine + cytarabine), limited availability of matched donors (hematopoietic stem cell transplantation), or the high relapse rate (MAPK inhibitors when used as single drugs).

- A standard of care for patients who fail front-line therapy (suboptimal response, disease progression or relapse) but the disease is not life-threatening (low risk LCH), remains to be established. Controlled prospective trials with appropriate endpoints (prevention of subsequent relapses and permanent consequences, as well as, improvement of quality of life) are still lacking.

- The same is true for some specific or rare clinical scenarios, i.e. isolated destructive pulmonary LCH, sclerosing cholangitis, LCH reactivation presenting with isolated diabetes insipidus, CNS-LCH of neurodegenerative type.

A currently ongoing international trial of the Histiocyte Society (LCH-IV International Collaborative Treatment Protocol for Children and Adolescents with Langerhans Cell Histiocytosis; NCT02205762) with a complex design (5 interventional and 2 observational strata) is looking for improvement of relapse-free survival and quality of life by targeting still unsolved clinical issues [56, 64].

6.2.1 Front-line treatment

The combination of prednisolone plus vinblastine is the most extensively studied first-line therapy in pediatric-onset LCH [42, 57, 65–68]. The major advantages are its extensively documented activity, its favorable toxicity profile and good tolerability in children, and its moderate costs, which make this treatment applicable even in countries with limited health-care resources [56]. In 'high-risk' patients of the LCH-III trial, the prednisolone plus vinblastine combination has induced response in risk organs in 70% of the patients after 6–12 weeks of treatment, and resulted in an overall 5-year survival of 84%, and a reactivation-free survival of 73% [57].

This regimen is the current standard frontline therapy for pediatric patients with multifocal and multisystem LCH treated outside of clinical trials (**Figure 3A** and **B**). It consists of 6–12 weeks of initial therapy (oral steroids and weekly vinblastine injections), followed by a continuation therapy given to total treatment duration of 12 months. The continuation therapy consists of prednisolone (day 1–5)/vinblastine (day 1) pulses given every 3 weeks.

6.2.2 Second-line treatment options for non-risk LCH relapses

The role of systemic treatment and the most appropriate drugs and regimens for patients with non-risk LCH who fail frontline therapy, is less clear. In the majority of those cases, LCH is confined to skeleton, skin and pituitary, and does not influence survival [40, 69, 70]. Similarly, most relapses of LCH are confined to non-risk organs and are not life-threatening. Relapses of LCH, however, are associated with an increased risk of permanent consequences [40, 69, 70]. The belief that control of the disease will prevent subsequent relapses and, thus, related permanent consequences, prompts physicians to use systemic chemotherapy for 'low-risk' multisystem LCH.

Temporary disease control in patients with low-risk disease, particularly in those, who have a relapse after complete disease resolution, is achievable both by repetition of the front-line regimen, or by application of a number of other single drugs or drug combinations [40, 50, 64, 69–71]. Remarkably, none of the available options can prevent further relapses and permanent consequences in all patients. Therefore, second-line treatment of non-risk LCH should be preferably offered within controlled trials. Future trials seeking effective treatment for 'low-risk' LCH should focus on appropriate end-points such as quality of life, risk for and severity of permanent consequences, instead on control of active lesions or remission rates [38].

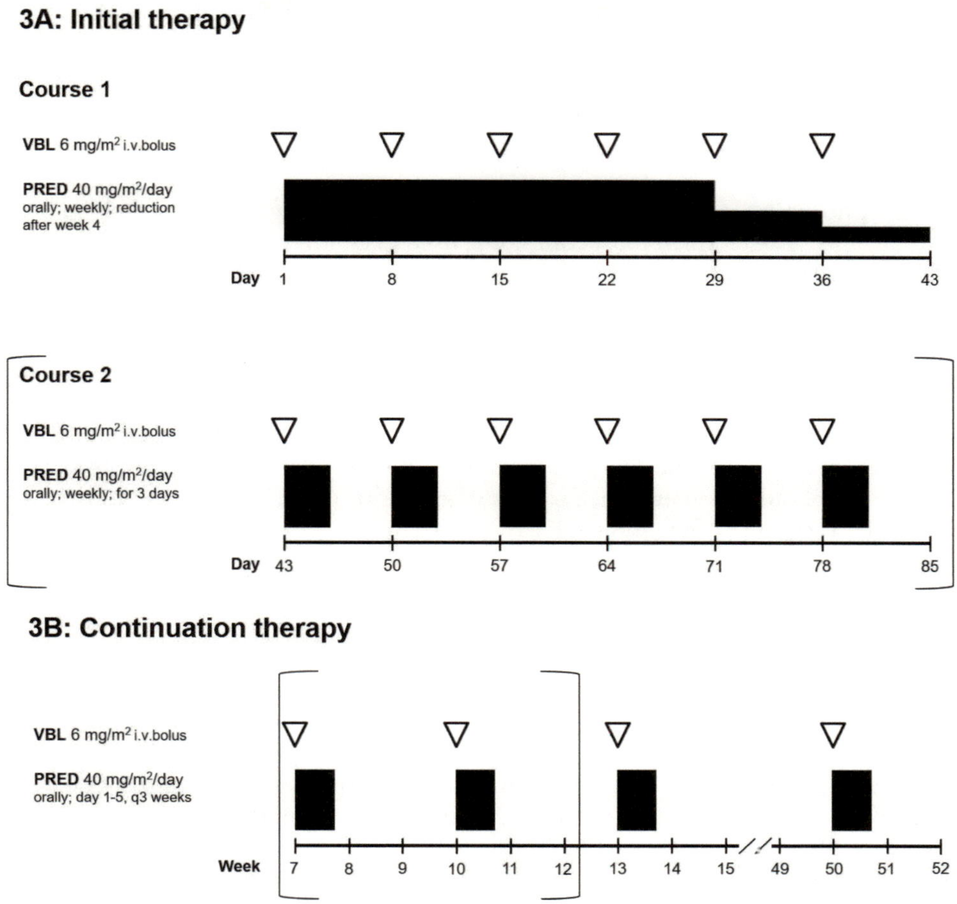

Figure 3.
Standard treatment of disseminated LCH.

Such trials are only possible within the frame of a large-scale cooperation and require implementation of innovative study designs and appropriate statistical methods.

For treatment outside of clinical trials, the following drugs and regimens seem to be reasonable choices, based on existing evidence for activity in LCH or experience from the clinical practice, as well as, justifiable toxicity:

- Patients with relapse months or years after stopping prednisone and vinblastine can benefit from re-induction of the first-line regimen [39].

- An alternative treatment regimen employs vincristine, prednisone, and cytosine arabinoside [72]. This regimen, modified for prednisolone duration, is being prospectively tested in the LCH-IV trial.

- Cytosine-arabinoside 100 mg/m2/das for 5 days every 28 days has been used with success both in patients with extracranial non-risk LCH and in CNS-LCH [51, 73].

- 2-Cholorodeoxyadenosine (2-CdA, Cladribine®, Leustatin®) at 5 mg/m2/day for 5 days per course has also been shown to be effective therapy for recurrent low-risk LCH (multifocal bone and low-risk multisystem LCH) with acceptable toxicity [71]. Use of 2-CdA should be limited to a maximum of six cycles to avoid cumulative toxicity and potentially long-lasting or irreversible cytopenias.

- Clofarabine is a proven effective therapy for patients with multiple relapses of low-risk or high-risk organs [51, 62]. In LCH, it is usually applied at a dose of 25 mg/m2/day for 5 days every 28 days for six cycles. Depending on hematopoietic toxicity or the need for longer treatment, (further) cycles at the same daily dose, but reduced to 3 days can be given.

- Bisphosphonate therapy has reported effects in treating recurrent skeletal LCH [74–77]. The regimen most commonly used in children consist of six doses of pamidronate at 1 mg/kg, given at 4-week intervals. Other bisphosphonates, such as zoledronate and oral alendronate, have also been successful in treating skeletal LCH in adults.

The choice of an individual drug or regimen requires consideration of comorbidities, previous treatments, cumulative toxicities and known individual intolerances and side effects. The decision remains on discretion of the treating physician, as the level of published evidence is not sufficient for a clear recommendation of a particular regimen or for a ranked list of preference.

6.2.3 Established salvage therapies for severe progressing multisystem LCH (very high risk LCH)

Two prospective trials have confirmed the curative potential of the combination of 2-CdA and Ara-C in patients with severe refractory to front-line systemic therapy MS-LCH [58, 59]. Unfortunately, this regimen is highly myelotoxic and associated with treatment-related mortality even if applied in experienced centers [59].

Allogeneic hematopoietic stem cell transplantation is another treatment option for very high-risk multisystem LCH with curative rate comparable to those achieved with the combination of 2-CdA and Ara-C [63, 78]. However, the most optimal conditioning regimen remains to be defined [78].

6.2.4 Toward rational treatment of LCH

The mitogen-activated protein kinase (MAPK) signalling pathway plays a key role in the regulation of gene expression, cellular growth and survival. A number of activating mutations affecting this pathway result in overactive downstream extracellular-signal-regulated kinase (ERK), which proves to be the ultimate driving event in LCH. Both specific inhibition of the mutated RAF and MEK kinases, as well as, downstream ERK inhibition (**Figure 4**) are undoubtedly appealing treatment options [49, 60, 61, 79].

The clinical experience available to date confirmed at least two essential expectations to BRAF inhibitors, namely in vivo activity and rapid clinical effect [80–83]. In patients with severe life-threatening LCH rapid clinical response is of particular importance. Currently published pediatric series show impressive rapid response to vemurafenib and prove that BRAF inhibitors can induce remission in patients with the most severe form of the disease [60, 61, 84, 85]. The clinical remission is sustainable as far as the treatment is given. However, most patients experience disease relapse shortly after treatment discontinuation. Hence, it is currently unclear whether treatment with a single inhibitor can eradicate the disease.

The European experience with vemurafenib in children with severe MS-LCH has shown that a daily dose of 20 mg/kg (2 x 10 mg/kg) is both well tolerated and clinically effective [60].

The major tasks to be addressed in controlled prospective trials are therefore: finding the most effective and least toxic specific inhibitors, establishing

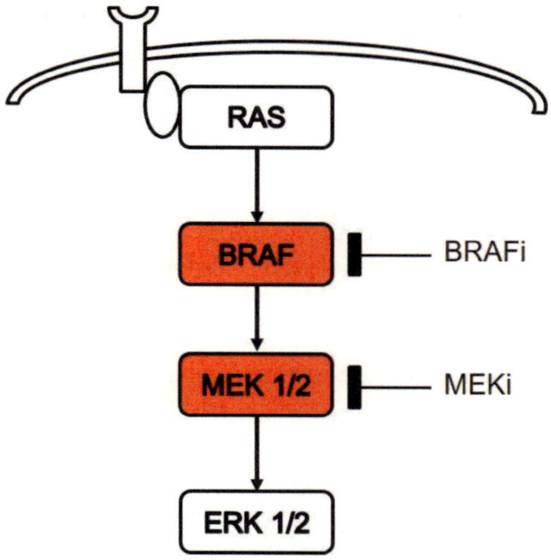

Figure 4.
MAPK pathway and relevant inhibition options.

downstream inhibition for patients without known mutations, defining appropriate pediatric dosages, and establishing optimal treatment duration and drug combination for a definitive cure.

6.3 Treatment of LCH of the central nervous system (CNS-LCH)

Treatment of the disease form referred to as a "non-granulomatous" or "neurodegenerative" CNS-LCH remains frustrating. The two currently recommended treatment options, monthly cytarabine pulses and/or monthly intravenous immunoglobulins have limited effect on disease course, mostly slowing down the process and achieving some improvement in anecdotal cases [33, 86–88]. A pilot study testing retinoic acid could achieve stabilization of the neurologic manifestations only [89].

A recently published paper has shed light on the underlying mechanism of the neurodegenerative CNS-LCH with possible therapeutic implications [90]. The authors could reproduce "neurodegenerative" LCH in a mouse model, by introducing the BRAFV600E mutation in the early erythro-myeloid progenitors, which give rise to the microglia. Moreover, in that model the neurodegeneration was preventable by BRAF inhibition. Human data are still limited and indicate that treatment with MAPK inhibitors can be effective if started in advance of irreversible brain damage [61, 91].

6.4 Treatment of other life-threatening complications of LCH

Apart of organ transplantation, effective treatments are still not available for the most severe disease-related complications of LCH, such as sclerosing cholangitis, and end-stage lung disease (honeycombing).

7. Current challenges and future directions

The current standard of care for pediatric onset LCH has been developed through laborious empirical trials over four decades. Future optimization of the treatment approach to MS-LCH and development of targeted drugs should be guided by biology insights. In the absence of this knowledge, the clinical needs have to be met by optimization of available treatments. The ongoing LCH –IV trial (ClinicalTrials.gov Identifier: NCT02205762) is designed to address the still remaining problems and unmet patient needs [46, 50]. The most urgent need is eliminating mortality (15–20%) among patients with risk MS-LCH. A two-step stratification based on risk organ involvement at diagnosis and lack of response to standard initial treatment (e.g. at week 6) allows for an early identification of patients who are at risk to die [50]. The combination of 2-CdA and Ara-C has proved to be curative, albeit too toxic. On the other hand, BRAF inhibitors provide rapid control of organ dysfunction, but alone are obviously unable to eradicate the mutated clone. A combination of the empiric and the targeted treatment options may be able to achieve ultimate cure, as this has been the case in other malignancies (e.g. Ph + acute lymphoblastic leukemia).

With all regimens used to date high relapse rates remain another unsolved problem in MS-LCH. Historical controls and preliminary data of the LCH-III trial have shown that treatment duration of 12 months significantly reduces relapse rates compared to 6 months of treatment [46, 57]. The question whether further prolongation of the total treatment duration will result in further reduction of the relapse risk is under investigation in the ongoing LCH-IV trial. A "2x2" factorial design will allow for additional evaluation of the role of oral 6-MP in the continuation treatment of MS-LCH.

There is an urgent need to address optimal treatment of some special disease presentations (i.e. new-onset central diabetes insipidus and non-granulomatous CNS-LCH. The potential of BRAF and MEK inhibitors is still insufficiently explored for these particular indications, but a mouse model delivers a rationale and awakes expectations [90].

Whatever new drugs and regimens appear appropriate testing in LCH, the design of the future prospective studies has to take into account the extreme clinical diversity and unpredictable natural course of MS-LCH, in order to avoid wrong conclusions and therapeutic strays [50, 56].

Acknowledgements

The authors are indebted to the medical student Martina Minkov for her assistance in the preparation of the figures.

Sigmund Freud University, Vienna, Austria provided financial support for the publication fees.

Conflict of interest

The authors declare no conflict of interest.

Author details

Katharina Sterlich[1] and Milen Minkov[1,2*]

1 Clinic Floridsdorf, Vienna Health Network, Austria

2 Faculty of Medicine, Sigmund Freud University, Vienna, Austria

*Address all correspondence to: milen.minkov@gesundheitsverbund.at

References

[1] Hand A. Polyuria and tuberculosis. Arch Pediatr. 1893;10:673-675.

[2] Schueller A. Ueber eigenartige Schaedeldefekte im Jugendalter. Fortschr Roentgenstr. 1915;23(1):12-18.

[3] Christian HA. Defects in membranous bones, exophthalmos and diabetes insipidus; an unusual syndrome of dyspituitarism: a clinical study. Med Clin North Am. 1920;3:849-871.

[4] Letterer E. Aleukaemische Retikulose.(Ein Beitrag zu den proliferativen Erkrankungen des Retikuloendothelialapparates. Frankf Zeit Pathol. 1924;30:377-394.

[5] Siwe S. Die Retikuloendotheliose - ein neues Krankheitsbild unter den Hepatosplenomegalien. Zeit Kinderheilk. 1933;55:212-247.

[6] Lichtenstein L, Jaffe HL. Eosinophilic Granuloma of Bone. Am J Pathol. 1940;16:595-604.

[7] Lichtenstein L. Histiocytosis X; integration of eosinophilic granuloma of bone, Letterer-Siwe disease, and Schuller-Christian disease as related manifestations of a single nosologic entity. AMA Arch Pathol. 1953;56(1):84-102.

[8] Nezelof C, Basset F, Rousseau MF. Histiocytosis X histogenetic arguments for a Langerhans cell origin. Biomedicine. 1973;18(5):365-371.

[9] Stalemark H, Laurencikas E, Karis J, Gavhed D, Fadeel B, Henter JI. Incidence of Langerhans cell histiocytosis in children: a population-based study. Pediatr Blood Cancer. 2008;51(1):76-81.

[10] Guyot-Goubin A, Donadieu J, Barkaoui M, Bellec S, Thomas C, Clavel J. Descriptive epidemiology of childhood Langerhans cell histiocytosis in France, 2000-2004. Pediatr Blood Cancer. 2008;51(1):71-75.

[11] Kaatsch P, Haaf G, Michaelis J. Childhood malignancies in Germany--methods and results of a nationwide registry. Eur J Cancer. 1995;31A(6):993-999.

[12] Salotti JA, Nanduri V, Pearce MS, Parker L, Lynn R, Windebank KP. Incidence and clinical features of Langerhans cell histiocytosis in the UK and Ireland. Arch Dis Child. 2009;94(5):376-380.

[13] Alston RD, Tatevossian RG, McNally RJ, Kelsey A, Birch JM, Eden TO. Incidence and survival of childhood Langerhans cell histiocytosis in Northwest England from 1954 to 1998. Pediatr Blood Cancer. 2007;48(5):555-560.

[14] Minkov M, Prosch H, Steiner M, Grois N, Potschger U, Kaatsch P, et al. Langerhans cell histiocytosis in neonates. Pediatr Blood Cancer. 2005;45(6):802-807.

[15] Bhatia S, Nesbit ME, Jr., Egeler RM, Buckley JD, Mertens A, Robison LL. Epidemiologic study of Langerhans cell histiocytosis in children. J Pediatr. 1997;130(5):774-784.

[16] Arico M, Haupt R, Russotto VS, Bossi G, Scappaticci S, Danesino C. Langerhans cell histiocytosis in two generations: a new family and review of the literature. Med Pediatr Oncol. 2001;36(2):314-316.

[17] Arico M, Nichols K, Whitlock JA, Arceci R, Haupt R, Mittler U, et al. Familial clustering of Langerhans cell histiocytosis. Br J Haematol. 1999;107(4):883-888.

[18] Ribeiro KB, Degar B, Antoneli CB, Rollins B, Rodriguez-Galindo C. Ethnicity, race, and socioeconomic status influence incidence of Langerhans cell histiocytosis. Pediatr Blood Cancer. 2015;62(6):982-987.

[19] Hamre M, Hedberg J, Buckley J, Bhatia S, Finlay J, Meadows A, et al. Langerhans cell histiocytosis: an exploratory epidemiologic study of 177 cases. Med Pediatr Oncol. 1997;28(2):92-97.

[20] Venkatramani R, Rosenberg S, Indramohan G, Jeng M, Jubran R. An exploratory epidemiological study of Langerhans cell histiocytosis. Pediatr Blood Cancer. 2012;59(7):1324-1326.

[21] Akefeldt SO, Finnstrom O, Gavhed D, Henter JI. Langerhans cell histiocytosis in children born 1982-2005 after in vitro fertilization. Acta Paediatr. 2012;101(11):1151-1155.

[22] Haupt R, Minkov M, Astigarraga I, Schafer E, Nanduri V, Jubran R, et al. Langerhans cell histiocytosis (LCH): guidelines for diagnosis, clinical work-up, and treatment for patients till the age of 18 years. Pediatr Blood Cancer. 2013;60(2):175-184.

[23] Ghanem I, Tolo VT, D'Ambra P, Malogalowkin MH. Langerhans cell histiocytosis of bone in children and adolescents. J Pediatr Orthop. 2003;23(1):124-130.

[24] Lakatos K, Sterlich K, Pötschger U, Thiem E, Hutter C, Prosch H, et al. Langerhans Cell Histiocytosis of the Orbit: Spectrum of Clinical and Imaging Findings. J Pediatr. 2020;230:174-181.

[25] Krooks J, Minkov M, Weatherall AG. Langerhans cell histiocytosis in children: History, classification, pathobiology, clinical manifestations, and prognosis. J Am Acad Dermatol. 2018;78(6):1035-1044.

[26] Minkov M, Potschger U, Grois N, Gadner H, Dworzak MN. Bone marrow assessment in Langerhans cell histiocytosis. Pediatr Blood Cancer. 2007;49(5):694-698.

[27] Berres ML, Lim KP, Peters T, Price J, Takizawa H, Salmon H, et al. BRAF-V600E expression in precursor versus differentiated dendritic cells defines clinically distinct LCH risk groups. J Exp Med. 2014;211(4):669-683.

[28] Braier J, Ciocca M, Latella A, de Davila MG, Drajer M, Imventarza O. Cholestasis, sclerosing cholangitis, and liver transplantation in Langerhans cell Histiocytosis. Med Pediatr Oncol. 2002;38(3):178-182.

[29] Ronceray L, Potschger U, Janka G, Gadner H, Minkov M, German Society for Pediatric H, et al. Pulmonary involvement in pediatric-onset multisystem Langerhans cell histiocytosis: effect on course and outcome. J Pediatr. 2012;161(1):129-33 e1-3.

[30] Yoon HS, Lee JH, Michlitsch J, Garcia-Carega M, Jeng M. Langerhans Cell Histiocytosis of the Gastrointestinal Tract: Evidence for Risk Organ Status. J Pediatr. 2019;212:66-72.e3.

[31] Lakatos K, Herbruggen H, Potschger U, Prosch H, Minkov M. Radiological features of thymic langerhans cell histiocytosis. Pediatr Blood Cancer. 2013;60(11):E143–E145.

[32] Grois N, Fahrner B, Arceci RJ, Henter JI, McClain K, Lassmann H, et al. Central nervous system disease in Langerhans cell histiocytosis. J Pediatr. 2010;156(6):873-81, 81 e1.

[33] Yeh EA, Greenberg J, Abla O, Longoni G, Diamond E, Hermiston M, et al. Evaluation and treatment of Langerhans cell histiocytosis patients with central nervous system

abnormalities: Current views and new vistas. Pediatr Blood Cancer. 2018;65(1).

[34] Komp DM. Concepts in staging and clinical studies for treatment of Langerhans' cell histiocytosis. Semin Oncol. 1991;18(1):18-23.

[35] Lahey ME. Prognostic factors in histiocytosis X. Am J Pediatr Hematol Oncol. 1981;3(1):57-60.

[36] Lavin PT, Osband ME. Evaluating the role of therapy in histiocytosis-X. Clinical studies, staging, and scoring. Hematol Oncol Clin North Am. 1987;1(1):35-47.

[37] Minkov M, Grois N, Heitger A, Potschger U, Westermeier T, Gadner H. Response to initial treatment of multisystem Langerhans cell histiocytosis: an important prognostic indicator. Med Pediatr Oncol. 2002;39(6):581-585.

[38] Minkov M. Langerhans cell histiocytosis: pragmatic empirism on the road to rational cure. Expert Opin Pharmacother. 2012.

[39] Titgemeyer C, Grois N, Minkov M, Flucher-Wolfram B, Gatterer-Menz I, Gadner H. Pattern and course of single-system disease in Langerhans cell histiocytosis data from the DAL-HX 83- and 90-study. Med Pediatr Oncol. 2001;37(2):108-114.

[40] Minkov M, Steiner M, Potschger U, Arico M, Braier J, Donadieu J, et al. Reactivations in multisystem Langerhans cell histiocytosis: data of the international LCH registry. J Pediatr. 2008;153(5):700-5, 5 e1-2.

[41] Lahey E. Histiocytosis x--an analysis of prognostic factors. J Pediatr. 1975;87(2):184-189.

[42] Gadner H, Grois N, Potschger U, Minkov M, Arico M, Braier J, et al. Improved outcome in multisystem Langerhans cell histiocytosis is associated with therapy intensification. Blood. 2008;111(5):2556-2562.

[43] Braier J, Chantada G, Rosso D, Bernaldez P, Amaral D, Latella A, et al. Langerhans cell histiocytosis: retrospective evaluation of 123 patients at a single institution. Pediatric hematology and oncology. 1999;16(5):377-385.

[44] Gadner H, Grois N, Arico M, Broadbent V, Ceci A, Jakobson A, et al. A randomized trial of treatment for multisystem Langerhans' cell histiocytosis. J Pediatr. 2001;138(5):728-734.

[45] Morimoto A, Shioda Y, Imamura T, Kudo K, Kawaguchi H, Sakashita K, et al. Intensified and prolonged therapy comprising cytarabine, vincristine and prednisolone improves outcome in patients with multisystem Langerhans cell histiocytosis: results of the Japan Langerhans Cell Histiocytosis Study Group-02 Protocol Study. Int J Hematol. 2016;104(1):99-109.

[46] Minkov M. An update on the treatment of pediatric-onset Langerhans cell histiocytosis through pharmacotherapy. Expert Opin Pharmacother. 2018;19(3):233-242.

[47] Donadieu J, Piguet C, Bernard F, Barkaoui M, Ouache M, Bertrand Y, et al. A new clinical score for disease activity in Langerhans cell histiocytosis. Pediatr Blood Cancer. 2004;43(7):770-776.

[48] Broadbent V, Gadner H, Komp DM, Ladisch S. Histiocytosis syndromes in children: II. Approach to the clinical and laboratory evaluation of children with Langerhans cell histiocytosis. Clinical Writing Group of the Histiocyte Society. Med Pediatr Oncol. 1989;17(6):492-495.

[49] Rodriguez-Galindo C, Allen CE. Langerhans cell histiocytosis. Blood. 2020;135(16):1319-1331.

[50] Minkov M. Multisystem Langerhans cell histiocytosis in children: current treatment and future directions. Paediatr Drugs. 2011;13(2):75-86.

[51] Allen CE, Ladisch S, McClain KL. How I treat Langerhans cell histiocytosis. Blood. 2015;126(1):26-35.

[52] Cohen M, Zornoza J, Cangir A, Murray JA, Wallace S. Direct injection of methylprednisolone sodium succinate in the treatment of solitary eosinophilic granuloma of bone: a report of 9 cases. Radiology. 1980;136(2):289-293.

[53] Egeler RM, Thompson RC, Jr., Voute PA, Nesbit ME, Jr. Intralesional infiltration of corticosteroids in localized Langerhans' cell histiocytosis. J Pediatr Orthop. 1992;12(6):811-814.

[54] Arceci RJ, Brenner MK, Pritchard J. Controversies and new approaches to treatment of Langerhans cell histiocytosis. Hematol Oncol Clin North Am. 1998;12(2):339-357.

[55] Broadbent V, Gadner H. Current therapy for Langerhans cell histiocytosis. Hematol Oncol Clin North Am. 1998;12(2):327-338.

[56] Minkov M, Rodriguez-Galindo C. Treatment of Langerhans cell histiocytosis: it is time to learn from the past. Br J Haematol. 2015;171(1):148-149.

[57] Gadner H, Minkov M, Grois N, Potschger U, Thiem E, Arico M, et al. Therapy prolongation improves outcome in multisystem Langerhans cell histiocytosis. Blood. 2013;121(25):5006-5014.

[58] Bernard F, Thomas C, Bertrand Y, Munzer M, Landman Parker J, Ouache M, et al. Multi-centre pilot study of 2-chlorodeoxyadenosine and cytosine arabinoside combined chemotherapy in refractory Langerhans cell histiocytosis with haematological dysfunction. Eur J Cancer. 2005;41(17):2682-2689.

[59] Donadieu J, Bernard F, van Noesel M, Barkaoui M, Bardet O, Mura R, et al. Cladribine and cytarabine in refractory multisystem Langerhans cell histiocytosis: results of an international phase 2 study. Blood. 2015;126(12):1415-1423.

[60] Donadieu J, Larabi IA, Tardieu M, Visser J, Hutter C, Sieni E, et al. Vemurafenib for Refractory Multisystem Langerhans Cell Histiocytosis in Children: An International Observational Study. J Clin Oncol. 2019;37(31):2857-2865.

[61] Eckstein OS, Visser J, Rodriguez-Galindo C, Allen CE, Group N-LS. Clinical responses and persistent BRAF V600E(+) blood cells in children with LCH treated with MAPK pathway inhibition. Blood. 2019;133(15):1691-1694.

[62] Rodriguez-Galindo C, Jeng M, Khuu P, McCarville MB, Jeha S. Clofarabine in refractory Langerhans cell histiocytosis. Pediatr Blood Cancer. 2008;51(5):703-706.

[63] Steiner M, Matthes-Martin S, Attarbaschi A, Minkov M, Grois N, Unger E, et al. Improved outcome of treatment-resistant high-risk Langerhans cell histiocytosis after allogeneic stem cell transplantation with reduced-intensity conditioning. Bone Marrow Transplant. 2005;36(3):215-225.

[64] Monsereenusorn C, Rodriguez-Galindo C. Clinical Characteristics and Treatment of Langerhans Cell Histiocytosis. Hematol Oncol Clin North Am. 2015;29(5):853-873.

[65] Feldges AJ, Imbach P, Pluss HJ, Sartorius J, Wagner HP, Wyss M. [Therapy of juvenile disseminated histiocytosis X. First results of a prospective study at the pediatric

section of the Swiss Work Group for Clinical Cancer Research (SAKK)]. Schweiz Med Wochenschr. 1980;110(23):912-915.

[66] Gadner H, Heitger A, Grois N, Gatterer-Menz I, Ladisch S. Treatment strategy for disseminated Langerhans cell histiocytosis. DAL HX-83 Study Group. Med Pediatr Oncol. 1994;23(2):72-80.

[67] Lahey ME. Histiocytosis X--comparison of three treatment regimens. J Pediatr. 1975;87(2):179-183.

[68] Rigaud C, Barkaoui MA, Thomas C, Bertrand Y, Lambilliotte A, Miron J, et al. Langerhans cell histiocytosis: therapeutic strategy and outcome in a 30-year nationwide cohort of 1478 patients under 18 years of age. Br J Haematol. 2016;174(6):887-898.

[69] Morimoto A, Kobayashi R, Maeda M, Asami K, Bessho F, Imashuku S. Impact of reactivation on the sequelae of multi-system Langerhans cell histiocytosis patients. Pediatr Blood Cancer. 2008;50(4):931-932; author reply 2.

[70] Pollono D, Rey G, Latella A, Rosso D, Chantada G, Braier J. Reactivation and risk of sequelae in Langerhans cell histiocytosis. Pediatr Blood Cancer. 2007;48(7):696-699.

[71] Weitzman S, Braier J, Donadieu J, Egeler RM, Grois N, Ladisch S, et al. 2'-Chlorodeoxyadenosine (2-CdA) as salvage therapy for Langerhans cell histiocytosis (LCH). results of the LCH-S-98 protocol of the histiocyte society. Pediatr Blood Cancer. 2009;53(7):1271-1276.

[72] Egeler RM, de Kraker J, Voute PA. Cytosine-arabinoside, vincristine, and prednisolone in the treatment of children with disseminated Langerhans cell histiocytosis with organ dysfunction: experience at a single institution. Med Pediatr Oncol. 1993;21(4):265-270.

[73] Simko SJ, McClain KL, Allen CE. Up-front therapy for LCH: is it time to test an alternative to vinblastine/prednisone? Br J Haematol. 2015;169(2):299-301.

[74] Arzoo K, Sadeghi S, Pullarkat V. Pamidronate for bone pain from osteolytic lesions in Langerhans'-cell histiocytosis. N Engl J Med. 2001;345(3):225.

[75] Brown RE. More on pamidronate in Langerhans'-cell histiocytosis. N Engl J Med. 2001;345(20):1503.

[76] Farran RP, Zaretski E, Egeler RM. Treatment of Langerhans cell histiocytosis with pamidronate. J Pediatr Hematol Oncol. 2001;23(1):54-56.

[77] Morimoto A, Shioda Y, Imamura T, Kanegane H, Sato T, Kudo K, et al. Nationwide survey of bisphosphonate therapy for children with reactivated Langerhans cell histiocytosis in Japan. Pediatr Blood Cancer. 2011;56(1):110-115.

[78] Veys PA, Nanduri V, Baker KS, He W, Bandini G, Biondi A, et al. Haematopoietic stem cell transplantation for refractory Langerhans cell histiocytosis: outcome by intensity of conditioning. Br J Haematol. 2015;169(5):711-718.

[79] Chakraborty R, Hampton OA, Shen X, Simko SJ, Shih A, Abhyankar H, et al. Mutually exclusive recurrent somatic mutations in MAP2K1 and BRAF support a central role for ERK activation in LCH pathogenesis. Blood. 2014;124(19):3007-3015.

[80] Charles J, Beani JC, Fiandrino G, Busser B. Major response to vemurafenib in patient with severe cutaneous Langerhans cell histiocytosis harboring BRAF V600E mutation. J Am Acad Dermatol. 2014;71(3):e97–e99.

[81] Haroche J, Cohen-Aubart F, Emile JF, Arnaud L, Maksud P, Charlotte F, et al. Dramatic efficacy of vemurafenib in both multisystemic and refractory Erdheim-Chester disease and Langerhans cell histiocytosis harboring the BRAF V600E mutation. Blood. 2013;121(9):1495-1500.

[82] Haroche J, Cohen-Aubart F, Emile JF, Maksud P, Drier A, Toledano D, et al. Reproducible and sustained efficacy of targeted therapy with vemurafenib in patients with BRAF(V600E)-mutated Erdheim-Chester disease. J Clin Oncol. 2015;33(5):411-418.

[83] Hyman DM, Puzanov I, Subbiah V, Faris JE, Chau I, Blay JY, et al. Vemurafenib in Multiple Nonmelanoma Cancers with BRAF V600 Mutations. N Engl J Med. 2015;373(8):726-736.

[84] Heritier S, Jehanne M, Leverger G, Emile JF, Alvarez JC, Haroche J, et al. Vemurafenib Use in an Infant for High-Risk Langerhans Cell Histiocytosis. JAMA Oncol. 2015;1(6):836-838.

[85] Kolenova A, Schwentner R, Jug G, Simonitsch-Klupp I, Kornauth C, Plank L, et al. Targeted inhibition of the MAPK pathway: emerging salvage option for progressive life-threatening multisystem LCH. Blood Advances. 2017;1(6):352-356.

[86] Allen CE, Flores R, Rauch R, Dauser R, Murray JC, Puccetti D, et al. Neurodegenerative central nervous system Langerhans cell histiocytosis and coincident hydrocephalus treated with vincristine/cytosine arabinoside. Pediatr Blood Cancer. 2010;54(3):416-423.

[87] Imashuku S, Fujita N, Shioda Y, Noma H, Seto S, Minato T, et al. Follow-up of pediatric patients treated by IVIG for Langerhans cell histiocytosis (LCH)-related neurodegenerative CNS disease. Int J Hematol. 2015;101(2):191-197.

[88] Imashuku S, Okazaki NA, Nakayama M, Fujita N, Fukuyama T, Koike K, et al. Treatment of neurodegenerative CNS disease in Langerhans cell histiocytosis with a combination of intravenous immunoglobulin and chemotherapy. Pediatr Blood Cancer. 2008;50(2):308-311.

[89] Idbaih A, Donadieu J, Barthez MA, Geissmann F, Bertrand Y, Hermine O, et al. Retinoic acid therapy in "degenerative-like" neuro-langerhans cell histiocytosis: a prospective pilot study. Pediatr Blood Cancer. 2004;43(1):55-58.

[90] Mass E, Jacome-Galarza CE, Blank T, Lazarov T, Durham BH, Ozkaya N, et al. A somatic mutation in erythro-myeloid progenitors causes neurodegenerative disease. Nature. 2017;549(7672):389-393.

[91] Diamond EL, Durham BH, Ulaner GA, Drill E, Buthorn J, Ki M, et al. Efficacy of MEK inhibition in patients with histiocytic neoplasms. Nature. 2019;567(7749):521-524.

Chapter 5

The Immune System of Mesothelioma Patients: A Window of Opportunity for Novel Immunotherapies

Fabio Nicolini and Massimiliano Mazza

Abstract

The interplay between the immune system and the pleural mesothelium is crucial both for the development of malignant pleural mesothelioma (MPM) and for the response of MPM patients to therapy. MPM is heavily infiltrated by several immune cell types which affect the progression of the disease. The presence of organized tertiary lymphoid structures (TLSs) witness the attempt to fight the disease *in situ* by adaptive immunity which is often suppressed by tumor expressed factors. In rare patients physiological, pharmacological or vaccine-induced immune response is efficient, rendering their plasma a valuable resource of anti-tumor immune cells and molecules. Of particular interest are human antibodies targeting antigens at the tumor cell surface. Here we review current knowledge regarding MPM immune infiltration, MPM immunotherapy and the harnessing of this response to identify novel biologics as biomarkers and therapeutics through innovative screening strategies.

Keywords: Malignant pleural mesothelioma (MPM), Immunotherapy, Fully human antibody, Tertiary lymphoid structure (TLS), BCR repertoire

1. Introduction

Malignant pleural mesothelioma (MPM) is an aggressive neoplasm principally due to asbestos exposure with a poor prognosis and a median overall survival (OS) of only 14 months [1]. Heavy asbestos utilization during earlier decades in Europe is the cause of actual disease incidence [2] and, despite many countries have banned asbestos use in recent years, a peak of MPM incidence is expected for 2020s due to a long latency and delayed disease onset [1, 3–5]. On the contrary, other countries that still make use asbestos are very likely to observe a substantial increase of asbestos-related disease and MPM in the future. BRCA1 associated protein-1 (*BAP1*) protein is an important player in DNA repair mechanisms, cell cycle control, carcinogenesis and apoptosis and almost 60% of MPM patients have BAP1 mutation [6–13]. BAP1 mutational status determines the insurgence of MPM [9, 10, 12–15], and influences the response to chemotherapy [16] and patient' s clinical outcome [17]. When other gene alterations are coupled to BAP1 mutation, synthetic lethality approaches could be evaluated as therapeutic options [18, 19]. Other frequent mutations are in the genes NF2, LATS2, TP53, SETD2 and TERT promoter as recently reported and are associated with different histotypes of MPM with epithelioid, biphasic and sarcomatoid features [20]. MPM is characterized by a lack of early and specific symptomatology and few reliable biomarkers and screening tools are available causing a late prognosis. As we recently reviewed [21], current therapies in clinical practice consist of surgery, radiotherapy and chemotherapy and innovative therapeutic approaches are being explored. From this survey emerged that new therapeutic modalities and prognostic biomarkers are urgently needed in order to grant a fair chance of survival to all MPM patients. Here we describe the interplay of the immune system and MPM at the tumor tissue level and envision strategies to take advantage of it and derive novel fully human MPM-targeting antibodies to be used as biomarkers and for the design of novel immunotherapies.

2. Inflammatory response and carcinogenesis in MPM

MPM's development is intertwined with the inflammatory response provoked by asbestos exposure. Asbestos fibers and fluid enter the pleural space where they reach the outer pulmonary parenchyma inducing an inflammatory response [22]. Later steps see macrophage infiltration guided by the presence of the chemokine CCL2 generated by mesothelial cells in response to asbestos fibers contact. Reactive oxygen species (ROS) and nitrogen species are produced by macrophages that, together with already present nitrogen and oxygen species generated from iron particles associated with the fibers, create reactive and dangerous free radicals responsible for mutagenic events and genomic instability [23–25].

Normally, cells which suffer genotoxic DNA damage undergo PARP-dependent apoptosis. Despite that, an *in vitro* study [26] demonstrated that damaged human mesothelial cells could be rescued and skip apoptosis by TNF-alfa produced by macrophages and by other intracellular pathways activated in mesothelial cells, such as NFkB [26–28]. Conversely, TNF-alfa receptor knock-out mice are protected from fibroproliferative lesions when exposed to asbestos fibers [29]. In summary, among innate immune system players, macrophages contribute to genomic alterations as well as survival of mesothelial cells in a context of inflammatory response to asbestos fibers.

3. Immune cell infiltrate in MPM

3.1 Tumor-Associated Macrophages

Tumor-Associated Macrophages (TAMs) are the most abundant cells infiltrating the pleural effusions [30–33] and are associated with poor prognosis [32, 34, 35]. *In vitro* and *in vivo* experiments support TAMs as potential targets for MPM treatment. Chemokines released by mesothelioma cells such as CCL4, CCL5, CXCL12 and, in particular, CCL2, are chemoattractants for monocytes [36–38]. CCL2 concentration is particularly high in malignant pleural effusions with respect to benign lesions or lung adenocarcinoma pleural effusions [39, 40] and affects CCR2-expressing monocyte trafficking in MPM [41]. When recruited to MPM lesions, monocytes and macrophages switch to immunosuppressive cells under the influence of growth factors such as M-CSF, IL-34, MCSF [41, 42] and cytokines such as IL-10 and TGF-β released by MPM cells. Those cytokines act both on monocyte and macrophage development and activation but also exert autocrine feedback loop functions on MPM cells [42, 43]. Also, the macrophage checkpoint marker and "do not eat me" signal CD47 is found to be highly expressed in the majority of patients with epithelioid mesothelioma [44]. In mesothelioma, TAMs show an immunosuppressive phenotype, characterized by $CD14^{mid}CD16^{hi}$ expression, reduced phagocytic activity and increased IL-10 production [45]. In addition, in vitro co-culture of TAMs with MPM cells boosts tumor proliferation and concomitantly reduces sensitivity to chemotherapy treatment [41]. Pro-tumoral activity of TAMs is also evident in mesothelioma mouse models where the removal of macrophages reduces the number of tumor nodules, metastases and tissue invasiveness [46].

3.2 Myeloid-Derived Suppressor Cells

Granulocytes and neutrophils are also present in MPM microenvironment and recruited by CXCR2 or CXCL5 and CXCL1 chemokines, respectively [36, 47]. Also, polarization and phenotype of granulocytes are affected by growth factors from the mesothelioma secretome which increases their expression of CD11b, CD15 and CD66b markers. These cells function as Myeloid-Derived Suppressor Cells (MDSC) and negatively affect T-cell proliferation via the production and release of ROS [48]. Also, the presence of consistent neutrophilic infiltrate as well as high numbers of neutrophils in the peripheral blood is associated with poor prognosis in epithelioid mesothelioma [49, 50]. However, MDSC targeting in MPM is still debated and controversial and requires further investigations.

3.3 T-lymphocytes

$CD4^+$ and $CD8^+$ T-lymphocytes are present in MPM microenvironment but in lower numbers compared to macrophages [32, 51–53]. T-regulatory cells (Tregs) are also present in MPM tissue but are less abundant compared to other solid tumors [54]. Principal chemokines present in mesothelioma secretome involved in T-cell trafficking are CXCL12, CXCL10 and CCL5. CXCR3, the receptor of CXCL10 chemokine, is upregulated in mouse models of MPM [47]. CCL5 concentration is high in MPM patients' peripheral blood with respect to asbestos workers and healthy individuals [55] while its receptor CCR5 is expressed on T-cell infiltrating pleural effusions [56]. As discussed in the following chapters, T-cells activation and programming is determined by the presence of neo antigenic stimuli [57, 58] and immune checkpoint expression [59, 60] in specialized immune structures organized *in situ*.

4. Tertiary lymphoid structures in solid tumors and MPM: where the anti-tumor response begins

Secondary lymphoid organs (SLOs) are lymphoid regions wherein dendritic cells (DCs) present antigens to T-cells in a major histocompatibility complex (MHC)-dependent way acting an efficient adaptive response against cancer, requiring the migration of DCs from the tumor site to the SLOs [61]. Consequently, B-cells are also activated in the SLOs by CD4+ T-cells, begin to proliferate and form a secondary follicle that will be converted to a germinal center (GC). This process induces T and B-lymphocyte proliferation and differentiation into effector T-cells and memory B-cells (MBCs), respectively, that migrate into the tumor contributing to cancer cells elimination, unless unfavorable/antagonizing events or exhaustive signals are in place. However, studies on the role of the immune system in tumors revealed that anti-tumor mechanisms can take place also at the tumor site within organized lymphoid aggregates similar to SLOs [62] called tertiary lymphoid structures (TLSs) [63].

TLSs are also present in the stroma, at the invasive margin and/or in the core of different tumor types [63, 64]. TLSs are composed of a T-cell-rich zone together with mature DCs but also by B-cell rich-GC surrounded by plasma cells (PCs). Inside TLSs tumor antigens are presented to T-cells by DCs. and both T- and B- cells are activated, begin to proliferate and to differentiate to effector memory T helper (TH) cells, effector memory cytotoxic T-cells, MBCs or antibody-producing PCs [53, 65–69]. High numbers of CD8+ and CD4+ T-cells in tumors determine TLS density [70] and evidence indicates a positive correlation of TLS density on OS and disease-free survival in lung cancer [66, 70–72], colorectal cancer [73, 74], pancreatic cancer [75, 76], oral squamous cell carcinoma [77] and invasive breast cancer [65, 78–80].

Importantly, its prognostic value is independent of tumor–node–metastasis (TNM) staging in most malignancies suggesting TLS can induce a systemic long-lasting anti-tumor response. High endothelial venules (HEVs) similar to those that allow entry of lymphocytes into SLOs could be detected near TLSs [65]. In this context HEVs allow lymphocytes to enter into tumors. Therefore, therapeutic approaches that enhance HEV formation would be beneficial to improve anti-tumor immune responses. Tregs negatively regulate HEV formation and their absence in cancer murine models promotes T-cell activation and tumor infiltration, favoring the eradication of the lesions [81, 82]. Also other immunosuppressive cell types, such as MDSCs, regulatory B-cell (Bregs) and cytokines, like TGFβ and IL-10, play a part in the development of an immunosuppressive tumor microenvironment (TME).

Tumor-resident Tregs co-express high levels of CTLA-4, OX-40 and GITR compared to effector T-cells and In murine models of MPM, the combination of anti-OX-40 and anti-CTLA-4 antibodies has synergistic effect on CTLA-4$^+$, OX-40$^+$ tumor resident T-regs and contributing to a clear tumor regression when compared to single-antibody treatment [83]. Coherently with this point, combined anti-angiogenic and anti-PD-L1 therapies favor HEV and TLS formation in murine models of breast cancer and neuroendocrine pancreatic tumors [84] suggesting that a powerful anti-tumor systemic response by ICIs is sustained, if not triggered, by the presence of TLSs *in situ*. TLS heterogeneity among human cancers has been analyzed via a pan-cancer gene expression analysis of TME cellular composition on The Cancer Genome Atlas (TCGA) data and MPM, as well as lung adenocarcinoma and lung squamous cell carcinoma, display high expression of a 12-chemokine gene signature associated with TLS presence [85] suggesting TLSs are frequent, but also heterogeneous [86].

Seventy percent of MPM cases contain lymphoid aggregates and about 30% of them contain GCs [31]. These aggregates are functionally similar to TLSs, in which T- and B- lymphocytes are apart in two adjacent regions surrounded by HEV, as already shown for ovarian and prostate cancer [87, 88]. Intratumoral CD8+ T-lymphocytes in high numbers are an independent good prognostic marker for MPM patients [68]. Additionally, structural inter- or intra-chromosomal rearrangements and single nucleotide variants have been recently reported from mate-pair and RNA sequencing-based analyses on mesothelioma specimens predicting the expression of potentially-targetable neoantigens [58]. Moreover, some of these neoantigens bind patient-specific MHC and specific tumor-infiltrating T-cell clones are expanded as observed through TCR repertoire analysis [58]. Indeed, TCR diversity and mutation/neoantigen load are inversely correlated, but both active and suppressive TME immune components, such as Treg and CD8+ T-cells, were present and equally balanced suggesting a scenario where activated anti-tumor CD8+ T-cells are counteracted by pro-tumoral immune suppressive molecules and Treg cells [57] or activated CD8+ T and CD4+ T-helper cells displaying phenotypic markers of exhaustion like PD-1, TIM-3 and LAG3 [59].

5. The importance of B-cell infiltration in solid tumors and MPM

B-cell follicles in TLS from non-small cell lung cancer and ovarian cancers contain bona fide Ki67+ GC B-cells expressing the activation-induced deaminase (AID) gene, that codes a critical enzyme in somatic hypermutation and class switch recombination processes typical of immunoreceptor genes, as well as, of BCL-6, the transcription factor involved in the late stage of B-cell maturation [66, 89]. Additionally, the presence of CD38+ CD138+ PCs around the follicle is highly suggestive of antibody production *in situ* [90]. Indeed, micro-dissected follicles subjected to BCR repertoire analysis revealed clonal amplification compared to peripheral B-cells, supporting the idea that locally presented antigens can elicit specific B-cell responses in several malignancies [87, 89, 91–94].

Additionally, PCs isolated from dense aggregates in tumor stroma [90], produce anti-tumor antibodies of the immunoglobulin G (IgG) isotype *in vivo* whose mechanism of action has not been yet determined. One possibility is that anti-tumor IgGs produced locally increase antigen presentation by DCs and/or directly promote the activity of specific subsets of CD4+ T-cells endowed with Fcγ receptors (FcγRs) [95]. The presence of IgG deposits in TLS, the spatial organization of TLSs that may favor DC priming by locally produced IgGs and the observation that tumor-derived immune complexes increase the expression of the co-stimulatory molecule CD86 on DCs *in vivo* [87] suggest that these mechanisms take place. In favor of the latter are the results of a meta-analysis in a large set of human cancers showing that the prognostic effect of T-cells is generally stronger when tumor-infiltrating B-cells or PCs are present, supporting the hypothesis that a coordination between cellular and humoral adaptive immune responses is crucial for effective anti-tumor adaptive responses [96].

The role of B-cells and the association of B-cell rich TLSs with survival and anti-PD-1 immunotherapy response in sarcoma and melanoma have been recently established [97, 98]. Interestingly B-cells are the strongest prognostic factor even in the context of low CD8+ T-cells [97] in sarcoma and class-switched MBCs are specifically enriched in melanoma ICI-treated responders [99]. In murine models of MPM treated with immunotherapy, the presence of B-cells is essential for good prognosis, indicating that antibodies are generated and contribute significantly and essentially to the therapeutic effect [100]. Consistently, B-lymphocyte infiltration in MPM tissue positively correlates with prognosis [38] although variable in its extent [101]. Moreover clinical [52] and preclinical data on B-lymphocytes contribution to MPM prognosis suggest that they elicit an adaptive cytotoxic immune response rather than acting directly as antigen presenting cells (APCs) [100, 102]. In this respect MPM and other solid tumors share many similarities and provide a solid opportunity to develop novel immunotherapies via the identification of MPM targeting molecules in patients.

6. Immunotherapy in MPM

Immune checkpoint (IC) proteins, such as cytotoxic T-lymphocyte-associated antigen 4 (CTLA-4), programmed death 1 (PD-1) and PD-L1, are regulators of the immune system that preserve homeostasis and hinder autoimmunity in physiological conditions [103]. ICs overexpression in MPM keeps anti-tumor immune response in check contributing to the creation of a local immunosuppressive TME [31, 104]. IC inhibitors (ICIs), i.e. antibodies targeting ICs, are used as immunomodulatory agents to interfere with the CTLA-4/B7.1/2 or PD-1/PD-L1 axes thereby helping to overcome tumor-immune escape [95, 105, 106].

Recently, PD-L1 expression in MPM has been assessed on tissue microarrays using two different FDA-approved antibodies and 22–27% of cases were positive for PD-L1 (1% cut off) [107]. PD-L1 is expressed in a high proportion of biphasic and sarcomatoid MPM cases and its positivity >1% is associated with a significant 10-months reduction in median OS compared to PD-L1 negative tumors [108, 109]. Similarly, high PD-L1 expression (>50%) in epithelioid MPM patients correlates with shorter PFS (6.7 vs. 9.9 months) [108]. Despite its prognostic value [59, 60, 110], PD-L1 expression is not a valid predictive marker of response to anti-PD-L1 therapies for several tumor types [111, 112], including MPM [113]. Anti-PD-1/PD-L1 therapies were tested in different trials in MPM patients [114–121]. Combination of pembrolizumab with PPC in first-line treatment compared to pembrolizumab or PPC alone, is currently being evaluated in the phase III trial NCT0278417, while nivolumab is being investigated in the randomized phase III trial CONFIRM (NCT03063450) in comparison with placebo [119]. Durvalumab activity, a PD-L1 inhibitor, in combination with first-line CCP was tested in the DREAM study (ANZ clinical trial registry number: ACTRN12616001170415). This combination resulted in an ORR of 61% using mRECIST and 53% using iRECIST criteria and in a 6 months PFS of 71% (mRECIST). On the basis of these observations a randomized phase 3 trial will be started [122].

ICs expression is controlled at different stages of T-lymphocyte activation and variable in tumor cells. For these reasons, a combination strategy employing two different ICIs in addition to chemotherapy has been proposed to achieve a synergistic effect by overcoming immune-resistance observed in some MPM patients. Encouraging results observed for different ICIs in combination [113, 123, 124] prompted the investigation of the nivolumab plus ipilimumab combination in comparison to standard PPC alone as first-line option in the phase III clinical trial Checkmate-743 (NCT02899299). Checkmate-743 has clearly demonstrated the benefit of nivolumab in combination with ipilimumab in first line mesothelioma treatment and based on those results obtained approval from FDA from October 2020. On 22 April 2021, the Committee for Medicinal Products for Human Use (CHMP) adopted a positive opinion recommending a change to the terms of the marketing authorization for the medicinal product Opdivo (nivolumab) in combination with ipilimumab for the first line treatment of adult patients with unresectable malignant pleural mesothelioma in Europe as well.

At present, efficacy and safety of adoptive T-cell therapies, in particular chimeric antigen receptor-transduced T-cells (CAR-T), in MPM and other solid tumors are under investigation [125, 126]. CAR-T-cells directed against mesothelin (MSLN), a glycoprotein expressed on MPM and other solid tumor cells, with a limited presence on normal tissues [127], represent a promising therapeutic option [128, 129]. Recently, Adusumilli and colleagues reported the outcome of a phase I clinical trial, NCT02414269, [130, 131] on MPM patients with pleural metastases from lung or breast cancer treated with anti-MSLN CAR-T-cells. Of note, the inclusion of anti-PD-1 therapy was crucial to elicit clinical efficacy and avoid T-cell exhaustion since no patient had an objective response before pembrolizumab addition showing the importance of conditioning the immune suppressive features of the TME also in this therapeutic setting.

Pembrolizumab plus anti-MSLN CAR-T-cell combination showed the best clinical outcome with an ORR of 63% (10/16) and a DCR of 75% (12/16). No evidence of on-target, off-tumor or therapy related toxicities higher than grade 1 was observed. Although applied to a limited number of patients so far, CAR-T therapies against MPM have shown really impressive results highlighting the different efficacy for advanced cell therapies compared to small molecule drugs or antibodies. Recently, a comprehensive review about immunotherapy in MPM has been published [132]. However, the limited availability of therapeutic targetable antigens hinders the efficacy of CAR based strategies for MPM patients. More targets are needed for MPM treatment in the future.

7. Making a hot tumor microenvironment

ICIs effectiveness in MPM treated patients highlight the presence of potentially active immune cells *in situ that* if properly unleashed can elicit anti-tumor responses. However, to achieve this goal, TME must be modified in order to abolish/interfere with specific immune suppressive cues. Interestingly, Barsky and colleagues recently reported a case of a man with MPM treated with a combination of palliative radiation and immune-gene therapy (GM-CSF) [133]. The outcome of this treatment combination was outstanding, resulting in a so-called "abscopal effect".

The abscopal effect is observed when a localized radiation induces an anti-tumor response at distant sites. RT can trigger an immunogenic cell death (ICD) [134, 135] and can stimulate antigen-specific, adaptive immunity [136]. ICD sets the stage for anti-tumor immune responses which include the release of tumor antigens by irradiated tumor cells, the cross-presentation of tumor-derived antigens to T-cells by antigen-presenting cells (APCs), and the migration of effector T-cells from the lymph nodes to distant tumor sites, suggesting that irradiated tumors can act as an *in situ* vaccine if appropriate conditions are in place [137–139]. The overall incidence of the abscopal effect of RT alone is low with 46 clinical cases reported from 1969 [139]. Those poor numbers witness the insufficiency of RT alone to overcome the immune resistance of malignant tumors. Immunotherapy can lower host immune tolerance towards tumors, therefore the combination of RT and immunotherapy can amplify the anti-tumor immune response, a hypothesis currently under investigation in the trial NCT02959463 where adjuvant pembrolizumab after RT in lung-intact MPM patients is tested. In a murine model of MPM, the abscopal effect can be induced by local RT and enhanced by immune suppressive CTLA-4 blockade as infiltrated T-cells, both in primary and secondary tumor sites, are predominantly cytotoxic CD8+ T-cells while Tregs are reduced [140]. Those observations corroborate the idea that a systemic tumor response can be unleashed by a local treatment thereby modifying the features of the TME.

8. The quest for specificity in malignant mesothelioma: how can we fill this gap?

Adoptive cell therapies in combination with ICIs are showing promising results for MPM patients. Their specificity or preference of targeting is granted almost exclusively by the use of antibodies or their derived fragments that are directed to tumor specific/associated antigens. First attempts of therapy using murine monoclonal antibodies (mAbs) in cancer patients failed due to neutralizing antibodies generation and to mismatch with components of the human immune system. These results highlighted the importance of using human or human compatible/tolerable biomolecules and prompted the design of novel screening platforms to find them. Antigen unbiased screening methods (**Figure 1**) can be used to this end to test *a priori* the targeting ability of antibodies to cells postponing the identification of antigens to lead candidates only.

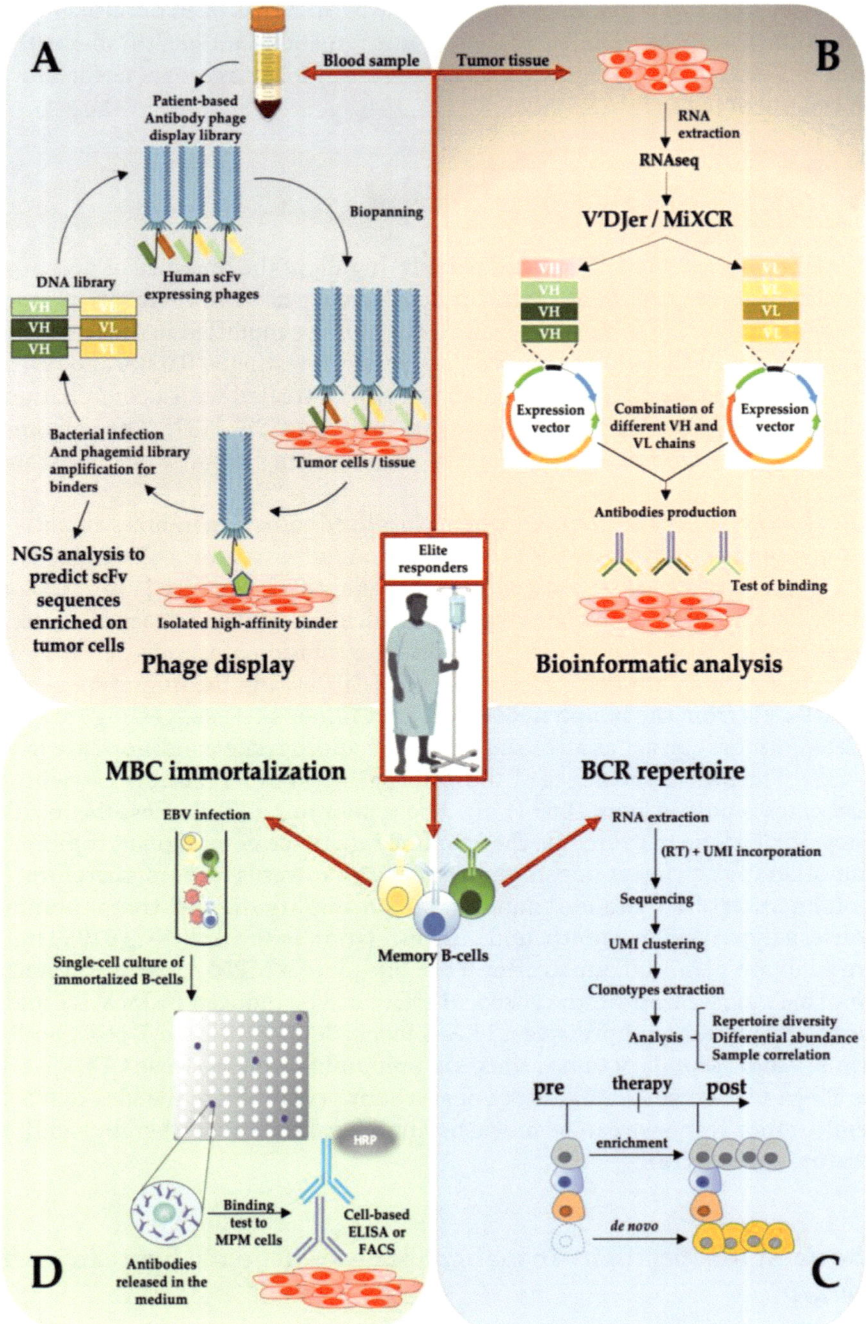

Figure 1.
Schematic representation of 4 antigen-unbiased screening strategies to obtain fully human tumor targeting antibodies. Panel ***A****: Patient derived scFv phage display libraries can be generated from MPM patient peripheral blood B cells. Those libraries are used to screen for novel specificities. Phage displayed scFvs undergo selection through consecutive rounds of panning on tumor cells to enrich for specific binders. NGS analysis allows the prediction of scFv sequences enriched on tumor cells. Panel* ***B:*** de novo *formed sequences, like those codifying the BCRs of infiltrated immune cells in tumor tissue can be retrieved using specific bioinformatic tools. Combinations of different heavy (VH) and light (VL) variable chains are used to generate candidate antibodies to be screened on cell or tumor tissues. Panel* ***C:*** *Analysis of BCR repertoire could be performed from memory B-cells from MPM patients. Enriched or de novo formed sequences could be monitored before and after a specific treatment in order to identify specific clones. Panel* ***D:*** *Memory B-cells from MPM patients can be immortalized through EBV infection and the immunoglobulins released in the medium of clonal cell cultures are tested on tumor cells by FACS or ELISA assays.*

9. From today's patients the future cures for MPM

As explained above, patients develop an immune response against MPM that, if unleashed, can be very effective. The presence of TLSs and the development of oligoclonal families of B-cells inside or at the border of MPM tissue are positive prognostic features and constitute a window of opportunity to capture human therapeutic antibodies. Now the next question is: how can we exploit this powerful reservoir of biologics to isolate or design targeting drugs? In other words: what technologies are available to take up this challenge?

10. BCR repertoire from sequencing data

Bulk RNA-Seq data from tumor tissue contain a hitherto overlooked picture of tumor and its ecosystem. Typically, data are analyzed to assess the expression of known transcripts, while *de novo* formed sequences, like those generated by T- and B-cells in the assembly and generation of their specific receptors, are usually disregarded since they fall off from the comparison with the reference transcriptome. However, these sequences can be retrieved from raw data and employed to extract the sequence of TCRs and BCRs from tumor tissue infiltrated immune cells using specific bioinformatic tools. One of them is MiXCR [141], a universal tool which takes raw sequencing data, including RNA-seq, as input and profiles TCR and BCR repertoires. As a reference, it uses a built-in library of V, D, J and C gene sequences from the human or mouse genome. MixCR output provides a list of clonotypes derived by assembling identical and homologous reads, corrected for sequencing errors.

V'DJer is another software that can process RNA-seq data for this purpose [142]. It can be run on BCR light and heavy chain data and employs unmapped paired end short reads aligning them against a reference transcriptome. Then, V'DJer detects VDJ rearrangements, generates contigs and quantifies the ones that represent the most abundant portions of the BCR repertoire. When the expression levels of BCR are low, there is an option to increase sensitivity of the algorithm at the cost of increasing the demand for computational resources. V'DJer has been used, for example, to retrieve antibodies from RNA sequencing data of melanoma patients from TCGA repository [142, 143]. At present, TCGA contains expression analyses of 87 MPM patients (TCGA-MESO) that could be used for this purpose. In addition, RNA can be obtained from FFPE samples containing TLSs in prospective and retrospective patients' cohorts.

It is possible to infer the sequence of resident B-cell clones by applying bioinformatic tools to RNA-Seq or by sequencing amplicons for immunoglobulin chains using specific sets of degenerate universal primers from whole tissue DNA or RNA/cDNA. The latter approach is implemented by the immunoSEQ platform (Adaptive Biotechnologies, Seattle, WA). In contrast to profiling using bulk RNA-Seq data, it is more precise since the experimental design is optimized to identify the BCR repertoire through the ImmunoSeq Analyzer software which is specific for this purpose. Its starting material can be both genomic DNA (gDNA) and cDNA: in order to assess clonal expansion of B-cells in tissues, gDNA is the best solution since each cell contains the same copy number, while mRNA transcripts can be very different among cells, depending on cellular activation and even the retrotranscription procedure can add other confounding factors. However, cDNA is a better choice if the goal is to find the most abundantly produced antibodies in situ, since there is a difference in the mRNA expression between activated and naive B-cells. Finally, independently of the method employed for their derivation, identified immunoglobulin heavy and light chain sequences can be assembled to produce candidate antibodies and test them for MPM target cells binding.

11. Memory B-cell receptor repertoire in MPM patients

A second powerful approach to obtain human antibodies targeting MPM cancer cells exploits directly the immune system of patients. Individuals exposed to viral agents, parasites and tumors develop an adaptive response against non-self and neoantigens. Anti-cancer treatments such as vaccines and ICIs elicit impressive clinical responses (reviewed in [95]) and an immunological memory in subgroups of cancer patients ("elite responders") has been reported. MPM is not characterized by high mutational burden [15] an important determinant of the response to checkpoint blockade.

The efficacy of the anti-PD-1 pembrolizumab was shown by Alley and colleagues in KEYNOTE-028 [116]. In addition, ipilimumab in combination with anti-TGFβ and anti-CD25 antibodies of syngeneic MPM in BALB/c animals resulted in: i) disease eradication in treated mice; ii) elevated levels of tumor-specific IgG antibodies in healed animals; iii) failure to regrow tumors in cured mice when re-challenged with the same tumor; iv) importantly, no response in the absence of B-cells, suggesting that antibodies generated upon treatment contribute significantly to the curative effect [100]. Besides that, CD20+ B-cells infiltration in MPM tumor tissue is a positive prognostic factor as previously discussed [38].

Therefore, the immune system of elite responders can be mined to isolate MBCs producing targeting antibodies. MBCs derive mostly from affinity matured and somatically hypermutated B-cells arising in the germinal centers [144] and constitute a reservoir of high-affinity antibody producers. These features make the MBC pool very attractive so biotech and pharma companies invest in the design of screening platforms to exploit it. For example, Oncoresponse, a company that developed a proprietary, clinically validated human-antibody discovery platform in partnership with MD Anderson Cancer Center follows this paradigm and identifies therapeutically relevant antibodies from patients showing elite response against cancer after immunotherapy. MBCs are easily accessible from the peripheral blood of donors and are suitable for viral immortalization to generate lymphoblastoid cultures for high throughput screens. MBC immortalization is usually performed by infection of peripheral MBCs by Epstein Barr Virus (EBV) [145] or by BCL-6/BCL-XL expressing vectors [146]. Those procedures generate cells that express BCR on the membrane and release their antibody into culture medium at the same time. BCR presence is exploited to isolate cells binding to labeled soluble antigens by cell sorting [146] so that subsequently immunoglobulin sequences from isolated cells can be cloned into expression vectors for large-scale antibody production. Companies like Humabs and AIMM therapeutics exploit those strategies to raise antibodies against specific targets. However, the same technology can be used to isolate targeting antibodies in an antigen unbiased manner as shown for melanoma via cell-based screenings of EBV immortalized B-cells [147]. In addition, human plasmablasts and MBCs can be cultured for a limited time using specific cytokines [147–152].

Importantly, these approaches to retrieve targeting antibodies do not rely on a prior knowledge of the target. Target identification in this case is postponed, initially drawing on the demonstration of efficacy and specificity towards MPM cancer cells. MBCs receptor repertoire can be obtained also from peripheral blood or draining lymph node purified MBCs by RNA-Seq mining for *de novo* formed or highly enriched variants after treatment in elite responders [142]. Advantages and

Approach	Antigen display	Advantages	Disadvantages
Phage-display technology with patient derived scFv antibody libraries	Antigen on cell surface	• Cheap instrumentation • Used with any cell type • Established technology • Fastest strategy to lead candidates • NGS driven selection of candidates	• Affinity maturation step is often needed • Reformatting in IgG format, if needed • Binding to normal human tissues to establish specificity *a posteriori*
BCR repertoire from the peripheral blood of elite responders pre and post therapy	Antigen on cell surface	• Availability of blood samples from elite responders • Antibodies are derived from affinity matured human immunoglobulins	• Possible downsampling • Cloning and production of candidate antibodies is required • VH and VL pairs are not known (unless single cell sequencing is used) • Requires a test of binding specificity to normal human tissues *a posteriori*
Bioinformatic analysis of BCR repertoire in tumor tissue	Antigen on cell surface	• Availability of large number of FFPE samples • Applicable to retrospective case series • Applicable to any RNA-Seq dataset	• Requires cloning and production of the antibodies • Possible downsampling due to low quality or limited sample material • VH and VL pairs cannot be known • Requires a test of binding specificity to normal human tissues *a posteriori*
MBC immortalization	Antigen on cell surface	• Easy availability of elite responder samples (blood/PBMCs) • Established protocols • Isolation of *in vivo* high-affinity matured and human compatible immunoglobulins • Basic technical expertise on viral manipulation	• Requires a BSL2 area • Identification of the antigens can be technically challenging • Requires a test of binding specificity to normal human tissues *a posteriori*

Table 1.
Advantages and drawbacks of antigen-unbiased screens to obtain fully human antibodies.

drawbacks of the different screening strategies for fully human antibody selection are summarized in **Table 1**.

12. Phage display screening using patient-derived scFv antibody libraries

A useful strategy to select human antibody fragments (Fabs and scFvs) against specific antigens or cells is phage display (reviewed in [153]). The importance of phage display has been restated in 2018 by the award of Nobel Prize in Chemistry to George P. Smith and Sir Gregory P. Winter"for the phage display of peptides and antibodies". Phage display has allowed the production of clinically relevant antibodies (reviewed in [154]). The presence of BCRs in TME, SLOs and in the peripheral blood of MPM and other tumor patients allows for the generation of patient derived scFv phage display libraries [155] that can be used to screen for novel specificities. Phage displayed scFvs undergo selection through consecutive rounds of panning on tumor cells to enrich for specific binders (**Figure 1**). Identified antibodies can be reformatted to fully human antibodies or used as fragments or building blocks for CAR constructs.

Importantly those antibodies will derive from the permutation of original VH and VL sequences of the B-cell repertoire during library preparation while for EBV immortalized cells VH and VL pairs will be the original ones as in the patient. Classically single bacterial clones were selected and grown to produce antibodies or phages displaying specific antibodies in order to test individually their targeting of a cell of interest. Nowadays, next generation sequencing provides an efficient, quantitative and quick analytical tool to assess the evolution of complexity of phage antibody-display libraries during consecutive biopanning enrichment stages. Phage clonal evolution during screening can be studied and used to identify putative candidate antibodies and promote their cloning and production for further testing their binding to cells [156].

An unbiased phage display approach has been used to identify tumor-targeting scFvs for both sarcomatoid and epithelioid MPM. In this study, 95 mesothelioma-targeting scFvs were identified and 21 candidates were characterized for binding by FACS and IHC and for their *in vitro* internalization capacity by MPM cells with the goal to deliver conjugated anti-tumor drugs directly inside tumor cells [157]. Further analyses identified MCAM/CD146 as one of the antigens. CD146 had been previously described as a marker in advanced melanoma [158] and other tumors [159, 160], it is expressed in all MPM histotypes and by a limited spectrum of normal human adult tissues [161]. The clinical utility of MCAM/CD146 detection in pleural effusion fluid and peripheral blood samples as a diagnostic and prognostic marker for MPM [162] is under evaluation. The generation of a phage antibody-display library from the entire antibody genes repertoire of a cancer patient has been also attempted. Rare cancer targeting antibodies have been identified by this strategy [163]. However, the immunodominance phenomenon typical of certain cancers [153, 164, 165] has hindered a wider use of this strategy in early attempts.

13. Conclusions

Despite amazing efforts made by the scientific community and the therapeutic options developed over the last decades, the discovery of a curative treatment for MPM is still elusive and constitutes an unmet clinical need. To-date, the most promising therapeutic approaches comprise immunotherapies and CAR-based therapies that have shown impressive although preliminary clinical results. The field needs to bet on and implement these novel approaches towards novel targets and antigens to cope with tumor heterogeneity and to provide effective treatments to be used in combination. The most innovative screening technologies for the generation of fully human antibodies are in place and combine elements from fields of science that started far apart and came together to serve the purpose. These include protein engineering, next-generation sequencing (NGS), virology and cell biology providing an opportunity to find novel and unknown therapeutic targets for MPM and cancer in general. Based on these premises, we believe that a future breakthrough in MPM management will come from the design of novel

ATMPs engineered to target antigens that are still unknown but that can be identified via unbiased screening strategies.

Acknowledgements

We thank Alicja M. Gruszka for her help in proofreading and editing this manuscript.

Conflict of interest

The authors declare no conflict of interest.

Author details

Fabio Nicolini* and Massimiliano Mazza*
Immunotherapy, Cell Therapy and Biobank (ITCB), IRCCS Istituto Romagnolo per lo Studio dei Tumori (IRST) "Dino Amadori", Meldola, Italy

*Address all correspondence to: fabio.nicolini@irst.emr.it and massimiliano.mazza@irst.emr.it

References

[1] Carbone M, Adusumilli PS, Alexander HR Jr, Baas P, Bardelli F, Bononi A, et al. Mesothelioma: Scientific clues for prevention, diagnosis, and therapy. CA A Cancer J Clin. 2019 Jul 30;69(5):402-29.

[2] Kameda T, Takahashi K, Kim R, Jiang Y, Movahed M, Park E-K, et al. Asbestos: use, bans and disease burden in Europe. Bull World Health Organ. 2014 Nov 1;92(11):790-7.

[3] Peto J, Decarli A, La Vecchia C, Levi F, Negri E. The European mesothelioma epidemic. Br J Cancer. 1999 Feb;79(3-4):666-72.

[4] Henley SJ, Larson TC, Wu M, Antao VCS, Lewis M, Pinheiro GA, et al. Mesothelioma incidence in 50 states and the District of Columbia, United States, 2003-2008. Int J Occup Environ Health. 2013 Jan;19(1):1-10.

[5] Beckett P, Edwards J, Fennell D, Hubbard R, Woolhouse I, Peake MD. Demographics, management and survival of patients with malignant pleural mesothelioma in the National Lung Cancer Audit in England and Wales. Lung Cancer. 2015 Jun;88(3):344-8.

[6] Cheung M, Testa JR. BAP1, a tumor suppressor gene driving malignant mesothelioma. Transl Lung Cancer Res. 2017 Jun;6(3):270-8.

[7] Yu H, Pak H, Hammond-Martel I, Ghram M, Rodrigue A, Daou S, et al. Tumor suppressor and deubiquitinase BAP1 promotes DNA double-strand break repair. Proc Natl Acad Sci USA. 2014 Jan 7;111(1):285-90.

[8] Carbone M, Yang H, Pass HI, Krausz T, Testa JR, Gaudino G. BAP1 and cancer. Nature Publishing Group. 2013 Mar;13(3):153-9.

[9] Affar EB, Carbone M. BAP1 regulates different mechanisms of cell death. Cell Death Dis. Nature Publishing Group; 2018 Nov 19;9(12):1151-3.

[10] Zhang Y, Shi J, Liu X, Feng L, Gong Z, Koppula P, et al. BAP1 links metabolic regulation of ferroptosis to tumour suppression. Nat Cell Biol. Nature Publishing Group; 2018 Oct;20(10):1181-92.

[11] Dey A, Seshasayee D, Noubade R, French DM, Liu J, Chaurushiya MS, et al. Loss of the tumor suppressor BAP1 causes myeloid transformation. Science. 2012 Sep 21;337(6101):1541-6.

[12] Bononi A, Giorgi C, Patergnani S, Larson D, Verbruggen K, Tanji M, et al. BAP1 regulates IP3R3-mediated Ca2+ flux to mitochondria suppressing cell transformation. Nature. Nature Publishing Group; 2017 Jun 22;546(7659):549-53.

[13] Bononi A, Yang H, Giorgi C, Patergnani S, Pellegrini L, Su M, et al. Germline BAP1 mutations induce a Warburg effect. Cell Death Differ. 2017 Oct;24(10):1694-704.

[14] Betti M, Casalone E, Ferrante D, Aspesi A, Morleo G, Biasi A, et al. Germline mutations in DNA repair genes predispose asbestos-exposed patients to malignant pleural mesothelioma. Cancer Letters. 2017 Oct 1;405:38-45.

[15] Bueno R, Stawiski EW, Goldstein LD, Durinck S, De Rienzo A, Modrusan Z, et al. Comprehensive genomic analysis of malignant pleural mesothelioma identifies recurrent mutations, gene fusions and splicing alterations. Nat Genet. Nature Publishing Group; 2016 Apr;48(4):407-16.

[16] Hassan R, Morrow B, Thomas A, Walsh T, Lee MK, Gulsuner S, et al.

Inherited predisposition to malignant mesothelioma and overall survival following platinum chemotherapy. Proc Natl Acad Sci USA. National Academy of Sciences; 2019 Apr 30;116(18): 9008-13.

[17] Farzin M, Toon CW, Clarkson A, Sioson L, Watson N, Andrici J, et al. Loss of expression of BAP1 predicts longer survival in mesothelioma. Pathology. 2015 Jun;47(4):302-7.

[18] Srinivasan G, Sidhu GS, Williamson EA, Jaiswal AS, Najmunnisa N, Wilcoxen K, et al. Synthetic lethality in malignant pleural mesothelioma with PARP1 inhibition. Cancer Chemother Pharmacol. Springer Berlin Heidelberg; 2017 Oct;80(4): 861-7.

[19] Zauderer MG, Szlosarek P, Le Moulec S, Popat S, Taylor P, Planchard D, et al. Phase 2, multicenter study of the EZH2 inhibitor tazemetostat as monotherapy in adults with relapsed or refractory (R/R) malignant mesothelioma (MM) with BAP1 inactivation. JCO. 2018;36 (15_suppl):8515-5.

[20] Quetel L, Meiller C, Assié J-B, Blum Y, Imbeaud S, Montagne F, et al. Genetic alterations of malignant pleural mesothelioma: association with tumor heterogeneity and overall survival. Mol Oncol. John Wiley & Sons, Ltd; 2020 Jun;14(6):1207-23.

[21] Nicolini F, Bocchini M, Bronte G, Delmonte A, Guidoboni M, Crinò L, et al. Malignant Pleural Mesothelioma: State-of-the-Art on Current Therapies and Promises for the Future. Front Oncol. 2019;9:1519.

[22] Donaldson K, Murphy FA, Duffin R, Poland CA. Asbestos, carbon nanotubes and the pleural mesothelium: a review of the hypothesis regarding the role of long fibre retention in the parietal pleura, inflammation and mesothelioma. Part Fibre Toxicol. BioMed Central; 2010 Mar 22;7(1):5-17.

[23] Park SH, Aust AE. Participation of iron and nitric oxide in the mutagenicity of asbestos in hgprt-, gpt+ Chinese hamster V79 cells. Cancer Res. Cancer Res; 1998 Mar 15;58(6):1144-8.

[24] Kamp DW, Israbian VA, Preusen SE, Zhang CX, Weitzman SA. Asbestos causes DNA strand breaks in cultured pulmonary epithelial cells: role of iron-catalyzed free radicals. Am J Physiol. American Physiological Society Bethesda, MD; 1995 Mar;268 (3 Pt 1):L471-80.

[25] Hei TK, Piao CQ, He ZY, Vannais D, Waldren CA. Chrysotile fiber is a strong mutagen in mammalian cells. Cancer Res. Cancer Res; 1992 Nov 15;52(22):6305-9.

[26] Yang H, Bocchetta M, Kroczynska B, Elmishad AG, Chen Y, Liu Z, et al. TNF-alpha inhibits asbestos-induced cytotoxicity via a NF-kappaB-dependent pathway, a possible mechanism for asbestos-induced oncogenesis. Proc Natl Acad Sci USA. National Academy of Sciences; 2006 Jul 5;103(27):10397-402.

[27] Yang H, Rivera Z, Jube S, Nasu M, Bertino P, Goparaju C, et al. Programmed necrosis induced by asbestos in human mesothelial cells causes high-mobility group box 1 protein release and resultant inflammation. Proc Natl Acad Sci USA. National Academy of Sciences; 2010 Jul 13;107(28):12611-6.

[28] Padmore T, Stark C, Turkevich LA, Champion JA. Quantitative analysis of the role of fiber length on phagocytosis and inflammatory response by alveolar macrophages. Biochim Biophys Acta Gen Subj. 2017 Feb;1861(2):58-67.

[29] Liu JY, Brass DM, Hoyle GW, Brody AR. TNF-alpha receptor

knockout mice are protected from the fibroproliferative effects of inhaled asbestos fibers. Am J Pathol. 1998 Dec;153(6):1839-47.

[30] Lievense LA, Cornelissen R, Bezemer K, Kaijen-Lambers MEH, Hegmans JPJJ, Aerts JGJV. Pleural Effusion of Patients with Malignant Mesothelioma Induces Macrophage-Mediated T Cell Suppression. J Thorac Oncol. 2016 Oct;11(10):1755-64.

[31] Marcq E, Siozopoulou V, De Waele J, van Audenaerde J, Zwaenepoel K, Santermans E, et al. Prognostic and predictive aspects of the tumor immune microenvironment and immune checkpoints in malignant pleural mesothelioma. Oncoimmunology. Taylor & Francis; 2017 Jan 20;6(1):1-10.

[32] Burt BM, Rodig SJ, Tilleman TR, Elbardissi AW, Bueno R, Sugarbaker DJ. Circulating and tumor-infiltrating myeloid cells predict survival in human pleural mesothelioma. Cancer. John Wiley & Sons, Ltd; 2011 Nov 15;117(22): 5234-44.

[33] Awad MM, Jones RE, Liu H, Lizotte PH, Ivanova EV, Kulkarni M, et al. Cytotoxic T Cells in PD-L1-Positive Malignant Pleural Mesotheliomas Are Counterbalanced by Distinct Immunosuppressive Factors. Cancer Immunology Research. American Association for Cancer Research; 2016 Dec;4(12):1038-48.

[34] Cornelissen R, Hegmans JPJJ, Maat APWM, Kaijen-Lambers MEH, Bezemer K, Hendriks RW, et al. Extended Tumor Control after Dendritic Cell Vaccination with Low-Dose Cyclophosphamide as Adjuvant Treatment in Patients with Malignant Pleural Mesothelioma. Am J Respir Crit Care Med. 2016 May;193(9):1023-31.

[35] Tanrikulu AC, Abakay A, Komek H, Abakay O. Prognostic value of the lymphocyte-to-monocyte ratio and other inflammatory markers in malignant pleural mesothelioma. Environ Health Prev Med. BioMed Central; 2016 Sep;21(5):304-11.

[36] Hegmans JPJJ, Hemmes A, Hammad H, Boon L, Hoogsteden HC, Lambrecht BN. Mesothelioma environment comprises cytokines and T-regulatory cells that suppress immune responses. Eur Respir J. European Respiratory Society; 2006 Jun;27(6): 1086-95.

[37] Li T, Li H, Wang Y, Harvard C, Tan J-L, Au A, et al. The expression of CXCR4, CXCL12 and CXCR7 in malignant pleural mesothelioma. J Pathol. John Wiley & Sons, Ltd; 2011 Mar;223(4):519-30.

[38] Ujiie H, Kadota K, Nitadori J-I, Aerts JG, Woo KM, Sima CS, et al. The tumoral and stromal immune microenvironment in malignant pleural mesothelioma: A comprehensive analysis reveals prognostic immune markers. Oncoimmunology. Taylor & Francis; 2015 Jun;4(6):e1009285.

[39] Blanquart C, Gueugnon F, Nguyen J-M, Roulois D, Cellerin L, Sagan C, et al. CCL2, galectin-3, and SMRP combination improves the diagnosis of mesothelioma in pleural effusions. J Thorac Oncol. 2012 May;7(5):883-9.

[40] Gueugnon F, Leclercq S, Blanquart C, Sagan C, Cellerin L, Padieu M, et al. Identification of novel markers for the diagnosis of malignant pleural mesothelioma. Am J Pathol. 2011 Mar;178(3):1033-42.

[41] Chéné A-L, d'Almeida S, Blondy T, Tabiasco J, Deshayes S, Fonteneau J-F, et al. Pleural Effusions from Patients with Mesothelioma Induce Recruitment of Monocytes and Their Differentiation into M2 Macrophages. J Thorac Oncol. 2016 Oct;11(10):1765-73.

[42] Cioce M, Canino C, Goparaju C, Yang H, Carbone M, Pass HI. Autocrine

CSF-1R signaling drives mesothelioma chemoresistance via AKT activation. Cell Death Dis. Nature Publishing Group; 2014 Apr 10;5(4):e1167-7.

[43] Fujii M, Toyoda T, Nakanishi H, Yatabe Y, Sato A, Matsudaira Y, et al. TGF-β synergizes with defects in the Hippo pathway to stimulate human malignant mesothelioma growth. J Exp Med. 2012 Mar 12;209(3):479-94.

[44] Schürch CM, Forster S, Brühl F, Yang SH, Felley Bosco E, Hewer E. The “don't eat me” signal CD47 is a novel diagnostic biomarker and potential therapeutic target for diffuse malignant mesothelioma. Oncoimmunology. Taylor & Francis; 2017;7(1):e1373235.

[45] Izzi V, Chiurchiù V, D'Aquilio F, Palumbo C, Tresoldi I, Modesti A, et al. Differential effects of malignant mesothelioma cells on THP-1 monocytes and macrophages. Int J Oncol. Int J Oncol; 2009 Feb;34(2):543-50.

[46] Miselis NR, Wu ZJ, Van Rooijen N, Kane AB. Targeting tumor-associated macrophages in an orthotopic murine model of diffuse malignant mesothelioma. Molecular Cancer Therapeutics. American Association for Cancer Research; 2008 Apr;7(4):788-99.

[47] Rehrauer H, Wu L, Blum W, Pecze L, Henzi T, Serre-Beinier V, et al. How asbestos drives the tissue towards tumors: YAP activation, macrophage and mesothelial precursor recruitment, RNA editing, and somatic mutations. Oncogene. Nature Publishing Group; 2018 May;37(20):2645-59.

[48] Khanna S, Graef S, Mussai F, Thomas A, Wali N, Yenidunya BG, et al. Tumor-Derived GM-CSF Promotes Granulocyte Immunosuppression in Mesothelioma Patients. Clin Cancer Res. American Association for Cancer Research; 2018 Jun 15;24(12):2859-72.

[49] Kao SCH, Pavlakis N, Harvie R, Vardy JL, Boyer MJ, van Zandwijk N, et al. High blood neutrophil-to-lymphocyte ratio is an indicator of poor prognosis in malignant mesothelioma patients undergoing systemic therapy. Clin Cancer Res. American Association for Cancer Research; 2010 Dec 1;16(23): 5805-13.

[50] Chee SJ, Lopez M, Mellows T, Gankande S, Moutasim KA, Harris S, et al. Evaluating the effect of immune cells on the outcome of patients with mesothelioma. Br J Cancer. Nature Publishing Group; 2017 Oct 24;117(9): 1341-8.

[51] Marcq E, Siozopoulou V, De Waele J, van Audenaerde J, Zwaenepoel K, Santermans E, et al. Prognostic and predictive aspects of the tumor immune microenvironment and immune checkpoints in malignant pleural mesothelioma. Oncoimmunology. Taylor & Francis; 2017 Jan 20;6(1):1-10.

[52] Chee SJ, Lopez M, Mellows T, Gankande S, Moutasim KA, Harris S, et al. Evaluating the effect of immune cells on the outcome of patients with mesothelioma. Nature Publishing Group; 2017 Aug 17;117(9):1341-8.

[53] Anraku M, Cunningham KS, Yun Z, Tsao M-S, Zhang L, Keshavjee S, et al. Impact of tumor-infiltrating T cells on survival in patients with malignant pleural mesothelioma. J Thorac Cardiovasc Surg. 2008 Apr;135(4):823-9.

[54] DeLong P, Carroll RG, Henry AC, Tanaka T, Ahmad S, Leibowitz MS, et al. Regulatory T cells and cytokines in malignant pleural effusions secondary to mesothelioma and carcinoma. Cancer Biol Ther. Taylor & Francis; 2005 Mar;4(3):342-6.

[55] Comar M, Zanotta N, Bonotti A, Tognon M, Negro C, Cristaudo A, et al. Increased levels of C-C chemokine RANTES in asbestos exposed workers and in malignant mesothelioma patients

from an hyperendemic area. PLOS ONE. Public Library of Science; 2014;9(8): e104848.

[56] Davidson B, Dong HP, Holth A, Berner A, Risberg B. Chemokine receptors are infrequently expressed in malignant and benign mesothelial cells. Am J Clin Pathol. 2007 May;127(5): 752-9.

[57] Kiyotani K, Park J-H, Inoue H, Husain A, Olugbile S, Zewde M, et al. Integrated analysis of somatic mutations and immune microenvironment in malignant pleural mesothelioma. Oncoimmunology. Taylor & Francis; 2017;6(2):e1278330.

[58] Mansfield AS, Peikert T, Smadbeck JB, Udell JBM, Garcia-Rivera E, Elsbernd L, et al. Neoantigenic Potential of Complex Chromosomal Rearrangements in Mesothelioma. J Thorac Oncol. 2019 Feb;14(2): 276-87.

[59] Marcq E, Waele JD, Audenaerde JV, Lion E, Santermans E, Hens N, et al. Abundant expression of TIM-3, LAG-3, PD-1 and PD-L1 as immunotherapy checkpoint targets in effusions of mesothelioma patients. Oncotarget. 2017 Oct 27;8(52):89722-35.

[60] Cedrés S, Ponce-Aix S, Zugazagoitia J, Sansano I, Enguita A, Navarro-Mendivil A, et al. Analysis of expression of programmed cell death 1 ligand 1 (PD-L1) in malignant pleural mesothelioma (MPM). Gangopadhyay N, editor. PLOS ONE. 2015;10(3):e0121071.

[61] Mellman I, Coukos G, Dranoff G. Cancer immunotherapy comes of age. Nature. 2011;480(7378):480-9.

[62] Drayton DL, Liao S, Mounzer RH, Ruddle NH. Lymphoid organ development: from ontogeny to neogenesis. Nat Immunol. 2006;7(4):344-53.

[63] Dieu-Nosjean M-C, Giraldo NA, Kaplon H, Germain C, Fridman WH, Sautès-Fridman C. Tertiary lymphoid structures, drivers of the anti-tumor responses in human cancers. Immunol Rev. John Wiley & Sons, Ltd (10.1111); 2016 May;271(1):260-75.

[64] Sautès-Fridman C, Lawand M, Giraldo NA, Kaplon H, Germain C, Fridman WH, et al. Tertiary Lymphoid Structures in Cancers: Prognostic Value, Regulation, and Manipulation for Therapeutic Intervention. Front Immunol. 2016 Oct 3;7(27):4410-1.

[65] Martinet L, Garrido I, Filleron T, Le Guellec S, Bellard E, Fournie JJ, et al. Human Solid Tumors Contain High Endothelial Venules: Association with T- and B-Lymphocyte Infiltration and Favorable Prognosis in Breast Cancer. Cancer Res. 2011 Aug 30;71(17):5678-87.

[66] Germain C, Gnjatic S, Tamzalit F, Knockaert S, Remark R, Goc J, et al. Presence of B Cells in Tertiary Lymphoid Structures Is Associated with a Protective Immunity in Patients with Lung Cancer. Am J Respir Crit Care Med. 2014 Apr;189(7):832-44.

[67] Ettinger DS, Wood DE, Akerley W, Bazhenova LA, Borghaei H, Camidge DR, et al. NCCN Guidelines Insights: Malignant Pleural Mesothelioma, Version 3.2016. Vol. 14, Journal of the National Comprehensive Cancer Network : JNCCN. 2016. pp. 825-36.

[68] Yamada N, Oizumi S, Kikuchi E, Shinagawa N, Konishi-Sakakibara J, Ishimine A, et al. CD8+ tumor-infiltrating lymphocytes predict favorable prognosis in malignant pleural mesothelioma after resection. Cancer Immunol Immunother. 2010 Oct;59(10):1543-9.

[69] Suzuki K, Kadota K, Sima CS, Sadelain M, Rusch VW, Travis WD, et al. Chronic inflammation in tumor

stroma is an independent predictor of prolonged survival in epithelioid malignant pleural mesothelioma patients. Cancer Immunol Immunother. 3rd ed. 2011 Dec;60(12):1721-8.

[70] Goc J, Germain C, Vo-Bourgais TKD, Lupo A, Klein C, Knockaert S, et al. Dendritic Cells in Tumor-Associated Tertiary Lymphoid Structures Signal a Th1 Cytotoxic Immune Contexture and License the Positive Prognostic Value of Infiltrating CD8+ T Cells. Cancer Res. 2014 Feb 2;74(3):705-15.

[71] Dieu-Nosjean M-C, Antoine M, Danel C, Heudes D, Wislez M, Poulot V, et al. Long-Term Survival for Patients With Non–Small-Cell Lung Cancer With Intratumoral Lymphoid Structures. JCO. 2008 Sep 20;26(27): 4410-7.

[72] Silina K, Soltermann A, Attar FM, Casanova R, Uckeley ZM, Thut H, et al. Germinal Centers Determine the Prognostic Relevance of Tertiary Lymphoid Structures and Are Impaired by Corticosteroids in Lung Squamous Cell Carcinoma. Cancer Res. American Association for Cancer Research; 2018 Mar 1;78(5):1308-20.

[73] Di Caro G, Bergomas F, Grizzi F, Doni A, Bianchi P, Malesci A, et al. Occurrence of Tertiary Lymphoid Tissue Is Associated with T-Cell Infiltration and Predicts Better Prognosis in Early-Stage Colorectal Cancers. Clin Cancer Res. 2014 Apr 15;20(8):2147-58.

[74] Posch F, Silina K, Leibl S, Mündlein A, Moch H, Siebenhüner A, et al. Maturation of tertiary lymphoid structures and recurrence of stage II and III colorectal cancer. Oncoimmunology. Taylor & Francis; 2017 Dec 20;7(2):1-13.

[75] Hiraoka N, Ino Y, Yamazaki-Itoh R, Kanai Y, Kosuge T, Shimada K. Intratumoral tertiary lymphoid organ is a favourable prognosticator in patients with pancreatic cancer. Br J Cancer. Nature Publishing Group; 2015 May 5;112(11):1782-90.

[76] Castino GF, Cortese N, Capretti G, Serio S, Di Caro G, Mineri R, et al. Spatial distribution of B cells predicts prognosis in human pancreatic adenocarcinoma. Oncoimmunology. Taylor & Francis; 2016 Apr 5;5(4):1-14.

[77] Wirsing AM, Ervik IK, Seppola M, Uhlin-Hansen L, Steigen SE, Hadler-Olsen E. Presence of high-endothelial venules correlates with a favorable immune microenvironment in oral squamous cell carcinoma. Modern Pathology. Springer US; 2018 Jun 7;:1-13.

[78] Gu-Trantien C, Loi S, Garaud S, Equeter C, Libin M, de Wind A, et al. CD4+ follicular helper T cell infiltration predicts breast cancer survival. Journal of Clinical Investigation. 2013 Jun 17;123(7):2873-92.

[79] Lee HJ, Kim JY, Park IA, Song IH, Yu JH, Ahn J-H, et al. Prognostic Significance of Tumor-Infiltrating Lymphocytes and the Tertiary Lymphoid Structures in HER2-Positive Breast Cancer Treated With Adjuvant Trastuzumab. Am J Clin Pathol. 2015 Aug 1;144(2):278-88.

[80] Savas P, Salgado R, Denkert C, Sotiriou C, Darcy PK, Smyth MJ, et al. Clinical relevance of host immunity in breast cancer: from TILs to the clinic. Nat Rev Clin Oncol. Nature Publishing Group; 2016 Apr;13(4):228-41.

[81] Colbeck EJ, Jones E, Hindley JP, Smart K, Schulz R, Browne M, et al. Treg Depletion Licenses T Cell-Driven HEV Neogenesis and Promotes Tumor Destruction. Cancer Immunology Research. 2017 Nov;5(11):1005-15.

[82] Joshi NS, Akama-Garren EH, Lu Y, Lee D-Y, Chang GP, Li A, et al. Regulatory T Cells in Tumor-Associated Tertiary Lymphoid Structures Suppress

Anti-tumor T Cell Responses. Immunity. 2015 Sep 15;43(3):579-90.

[83] Fear VS, Tilsed C, Chee J, Forbes CA, Casey T, Solin JN, et al. Combination immune checkpoint blockade as an effective therapy for mesothelioma. Oncoimmunology. Taylor & Francis; 2018 Sep 12;7(10):1-14.

[84] Allen E, Jabouille A, Rivera LB, Lodewijckx I, Missiaen R, Steri V, et al. Combined antiangiogenic and anti-PD-L1 therapy stimulates tumor immunity through HEV formation. Sci Transl Med. 2017 Apr 12;9(385): eaak9679.

[85] Coppola D, Nebozhyn M, Khalil F, Dai H, Yeatman T, Loboda A, et al. Unique ectopic lymph node-like structures present in human primary colorectal carcinoma are identified by immune gene array profiling. Am J Pathol. 2011 Jul;179(1):37-45.

[86] Sautès-Fridman C, Petitprez F, Calderaro J, Fridman WH. Tertiary lymphoid structures in the era of cancer immunotherapy. Nature Publishing Group. Nature Publishing Group; 2019 Jun;19(6):307-25.

[87] Montfort A, Pearce O, Maniati E, Vincent BG, Bixby L, Böhm S, et al. A Strong B-cell Response Is Part of the Immune Landscape in Human High-Grade Serous Ovarian Metastases. Clin Cancer Res. 2017 Jan 2;23(1): 250-62.

[88] García-Hernández M de LL, Uribe-Uribe NO, Espinosa-González R, Kast WM, Khader SA, Rangel-Moreno J. A Unique Cellular and Molecular Microenvironment Is Present in Tertiary Lymphoid Organs of Patients with Spontaneous Prostate Cancer Regression. Front Immunol. 2017 May 17;8:87-21.

[89] Nielsen JS, Sahota RA, Milne K, Kost SE, Nesslinger NJ, Watson PH, et al. CD20+ Tumor-Infiltrating Lymphocytes Have an Atypical CD27- Memory Phenotype and Together with CD8+ T Cells Promote Favorable Prognosis in Ovarian Cancer. Clin Cancer Res. 2012 Jun 14;18(12):3281-92.

[90] Kroeger DR, Milne K, Nelson BH. Tumor-Infiltrating Plasma Cells Are Associated with Tertiary Lymphoid Structures, Cytolytic T-Cell Responses, and Superior Prognosis in Ovarian Cancer. Clin Cancer Res. 2016 Jun 14;22(12):3005-15.

[91] Coronella JA, Spier C, Welch M, Trevor KT, Stopeck AT, Villar H, et al. Antigen-Driven Oligoclonal Expansion of Tumor-Infiltrating B Cells in Infiltrating Ductal Carcinoma of the Breast. JI. 2002 Aug 15;169(4):1829-36.

[92] Schlößer HA, Thelen M, Lechner A, Wennhold K, Garcia-Marquez MA, Rothschild SI, et al. B cells in esophago-gastric adenocarcinoma are highly differentiated, organize in tertiary lymphoid structures and produce tumor-specific antibodies. Oncoimmunology. Taylor & Francis; 2018 Oct 29;8(1):e1512458.

[93] Nzula S, Going JJ, Stott DI. Antigen-driven clonal proliferation, somatic hypermutation, and selection of B lymphocytes infiltrating human ductal breast carcinomas. Cancer Res. 2003 Jun 15;63(12):3275-80.

[94] Cipponi A, Mercier M, Seremet T, Baurain J-F, Théate I, van den Oord J, et al. Neogenesis of Lymphoid Structures and Antibody Responses Occur in Human Melanoma Metastases. Cancer Res. 2012 Aug 14;72(16):3997-4007.

[95] Darvin P, Toor SM, Sasidharan Nair V, Elkord E. Immune checkpoint inhibitors: recent progress and potential biomarkers. Exp Mol Med. Nature

Publishing Group; 2018 Dec 13;50(12):165-11.

[96] Wouters MCA, Nelson BH. Prognostic Significance of Tumor-Infiltrating B Cells and Plasma Cells in Human Cancer. Clin Cancer Res. 2018 Dec 15;24(24):6125-35.

[97] Petitprez F, de Reyniès A, Keung EZ, Chen TW-W, Sun C-M, Calderaro J, et al. B cells are associated with survival and immunotherapy response in sarcoma. Nature. Nature Publishing Group; 2020 Jan;577(7791):556-60.

[98] Cabrita R, Lauss M, Sanna A, Donia M, Skaarup Larsen M, Mitra S, et al. Tertiary lymphoid structures improve immunotherapy and survival in melanoma. Nature. Nature Publishing Group; 2020 Jan;577(7791):561-5.

[99] Helmink BA, Reddy SM, Gao J, Zhang S, Basar R, Thakur R, et al. B cells and tertiary lymphoid structures promote immunotherapy response. Nature. Nature Publishing Group; 2020 Jan;577(7791):549-55.

[100] Krishnan S, Bakker E, Lee C, Kissick HT, Ireland DJ, Beilharz MW. Successful combined intratumoral immunotherapy of established murine mesotheliomas requires B-cell involvement. J Interferon Cytokine Res. Mary Ann Liebert, Inc. 140 Huguenot Street, 3rd Floor New Rochelle, NY 10801 USA; 2015 Feb;35(2):100-7.

[101] Minnema-Luiting J, Vroman H, Aerts J, Cornelissen R. Heterogeneity in Immune Cell Content in Malignant Pleural Mesothelioma. Int J Mol Sci. Multidisciplinary Digital Publishing Institute; 2018 Apr;19(4):1041-12.

[102] Jackaman C, Cornwall S, Graham PT, Nelson DJ. CD40-activated B cells contribute to mesothelioma tumor regression. Immunol Cell Biol. 2011 Feb;89(2):255-67.

[103] Buchbinder EI, Desai A. CTLA-4 and PD-1 Pathways: Similarities, Differences, and Implications of Their Inhibition. Am J Clin Oncol. 2016 Feb;39(1):98-106.

[104] Pasello G, Zago G, Lunardi F, Urso L, Kern I, Vlacic G, et al. Malignant pleural mesothelioma immune microenvironment and checkpoint expression: correlation with clinical-pathological features and intratumor heterogeneity over time. Ann Oncol. 2018 May 1;29(5):1258-65.

[105] Nowak AK, Forde PM. Immunotherapy trials in mesothelioma - promising results, but don't stop here. Nat Rev Clin Oncol. 2019 Dec;16(12):726-8.

[106] Wei SC, Duffy CR, Allison JP. Fundamental Mechanisms of Immune Checkpoint Blockade Therapy. Cancer Discov. American Association for Cancer Research; 2018 Sep;8(9):1069-86.

[107] Chapel DB, Stewart R, Furtado LV, Husain AN, Krausz T, Deftereos G. Tumor PD-L1 expression in malignant pleural and peritoneal mesothelioma by Dako PD-L1 22C3 pharmDx and Dako PD-L1 28-8 pharmDx assays. Human Pathology. 2019 May;87:11-7.

[108] Brosseau S, Danel C, Scherpereel A, Mazieres J, Lantuejoul S, Margery J, et al. Shorter Survival in Malignant Pleural Mesothelioma Patients With High PD-L1 Expression Associated With Sarcomatoid or Biphasic Histology Subtype: A Series of 214 Cases From the Bio-MAPS Cohort. Clin Lung Cancer. 2019 Sep;20(5):e564-75.

[109] Nguyen BH, Montgomery R, Fadia M, Wang J, Ali S. PD-L1 expression associated with worse survival outcome in malignant pleural mesothelioma. Asia Pac J Clin Oncol.

John Wiley & Sons, Ltd (10.1111); 2018 Feb;14(1):69-73.

[110] Gennen K, Käsmann L, Taugner J, Eze C, Karin M, Roengvoraphoj O, et al. Prognostic value of PD-L1 expression on tumor cells combined with CD8+ TIL density in patients with locally advanced non-small cell lung cancer treated with concurrent chemoradiotherapy. Radiat Oncol. BioMed Central; 2020 Jan 2;15(1):5-12.

[111] Shen X, Zhao B. Efficacy of PD-1 or PD-L1 inhibitors and PD-L1 expression status in cancer: meta-analysis. BMJ. 2018 Sep 10;362:k3529.

[112] Conroy JM, Pabla S, Nesline MK, Glenn ST, Papanicolau-Sengos A, Burgher B, et al. Next generation sequencing of PD-L1 for predicting response to immune checkpoint inhibitors. J Immunother Cancer. BMJ Specialist Journals; 2019 Jan 24;7(1):18.

[113] Scherpereel A, Mazieres J, Greillier L, Lantuejoul S, Dô P, Bylicki O, et al. Nivolumab or nivolumab plus ipilimumab in patients with relapsed malignant pleural mesothelioma (IFCT-1501 MAPS2): a multicentre, open-label, randomised, non-comparative, phase 2 trial. Lancet Oncol. 2019 Feb;20(2):239-53.

[114] Calabrò L, Morra A, Fonsatti E, Cutaia O, Amato G, Giannarelli D, et al. Tremelimumab for patients with chemotherapy-resistant advanced malignant mesothelioma: an open-label, single-arm, phase 2 trial. Lancet Oncol. 2013 Oct;14(11):1104-11.

[115] Maio M, Scherpereel A, Calabrò L, Aerts J, Cedres Perez S, Bearz A, et al. Tremelimumab as second-line or third-line treatment in relapsed malignant mesothelioma (DETERMINE): a multicentre, international, randomised, double-blind, placebo-controlled phase 2b trial. Lancet Oncol. 2017 Sep;18(9):1261-73.

[116] Alley EW, Lopez J, Santoro A, Morosky A, Saraf S, Piperdi B, et al. Clinical safety and activity of pembrolizumab in patients with malignant pleural mesothelioma (KEYNOTE-028): preliminary results from a non-randomised, open-label, phase 1b trial. Lancet Oncol. 2017 May;18(5):623-30.

[117] Desai A, Karrison T, Rose B, Tan Y, Hill B, Pemberton E, et al. OA08.03 Phase II Trial of Pembrolizumab (NCT02399371) In Previously-Treated Malignant Mesothelioma (MM): Final Analysis. Journal of Thoracic Oncology. Elsevier Inc; 2018 Oct 1;13(Supplement):S339.

[118] Popat S, Curioni-Fontecedro A, Polydoropoulou V, Shah R, O'Brien M, Pope A, et al. LBA91_PRA multicentre randomized phase III trial comparing pembrolizumab (P) vs single agent chemotherapy (CT) for advanced pre-treated malignant pleural mesothelioma (MPM): Results from the European Thoracic Oncology Platform (ETOP 9-15) PROMISE-meso trial. annonc. 2019 Oct 1;30(Supplement_5).

[119] Fennell DA, Kirkpatrick E, Cozens K, Nye M, Lester J, Hanna G, et al. CONFIRM: a double-blind, placebo-controlled phase III clinical trial investigating the effect of nivolumab in patients with relapsed mesothelioma: study protocol for a randomised controlled trial. Trials. BioMed Central; 2018 Apr 18;19(1):233-10.

[120] Quispel-Janssen J, Zago G, Schouten R, Buikhuisen W, Monkhorst K, Thunissen E, et al. OA13.01 A Phase II Study of Nivolumab in Malignant Pleural Mesothelioma (NivoMes): with Translational Research (TR) Biopies. Journal of Thoracic Oncology. Elsevier; 2017 Jan 1;12(Supplement):S292-3.

[121] Okada M, Kijima T, Aoe K, Kato T, Fujimoto N, Nakagawa K, et al. Clinical

Efficacy and Safety of Nivolumab: Results of a Multicenter, Open-label, Single-arm, Japanese Phase II study in Malignant Pleural Mesohelioma (MERIT). Clin Cancer Res. 2019 Sep 15;25(18):5485.

[122] Nowak AK, Lesterhuis WJ, Hughes BGM, Brown C, Kok PS, O'Byrne KJ, et al. DREAM: A phase II study of durvalumab with first line chemotherapy in mesothelioma—First results. JCO. American Society of Clinical Oncology; 2018 May 20;36(15_suppl):8503-3.

[123] Calabrò L, Morra A, Giannarelli D, Amato G, D'Incecco A, Covre A, et al. Tremelimumab combined with durvalumab in patients with mesothelioma (NIBIT-MESO-1): an open-label, non-randomised, phase 2 study. Lancet Respir Med. 2018 Jun;6(6):451-60.

[124] Disselhorst MJ, Quispel-Janssen J, Lalezari F, Monkhorst K, de Vries JF, van der Noort V, et al. Ipilimumab and nivolumab in the treatment of recurrent malignant pleural mesothelioma (INITIATE): results of a prospective, single-arm, phase 2 trial. Lancet Respir Med. 2019 Mar;7(3):260-70.

[125] Zeltsman M, Dozier J, McGee E, Ngai D, Adusumilli PS. CAR T-cell therapy for lung cancer and malignant pleural mesothelioma. Transl Res. 2017 Sep;187:1-10.

[126] Martinez M, Moon EK. CAR T Cells for Solid Tumors: New Strategies for Finding, Infiltrating, and Surviving in the Tumor Microenvironment. Front Immunol. Frontiers; 2019;10:128.

[127] Lv J, Li P. Mesothelin as a biomarker for targeted therapy. Biomark Res. BioMed Central; 2019;7(1):18-8.

[128] Zhao Y, Moon E, Carpenito C, Paulos CM, Liu X, Brennan AL, et al. Multiple injections of electroporated autologous T cells expressing a chimeric antigen receptor mediate regression of human disseminated tumor. Cancer Res. 2010 Nov 15;70(22):9053-61.

[129] Zhang Z, Jiang D, Yang H, He Z, Liu X, Qin W, et al. Modified CAR T cells targeting membrane-proximal epitope of mesothelin enhances the antitumor function against large solid tumor. Cell Death Dis. Nature Publishing Group; 2019 Jun 17;10(7): 476-12.

[130] Adusumilli PS, Zauderer MG, Rusch VW, O 039 Cearbhaill RE, Zhu A, Ngai DA, et al. Abstract CT036: A phase I clinical trial of malignant pleural disease treated with regionally delivered autologous mesothelin-targeted CAR T cells: Safety and efficacy. Cancer Res. 2019 Jul 1;79(13 Supplement):CT036.

[131] Adusumilli PS, Cherkassky L, Villena-Vargas J, Colovos C, Servais E, Plotkin J, et al. Regional delivery of mesothelin-targeted CAR T cell therapy generates potent and long-lasting CD4-dependent tumor immunity. Sci Transl Med. 2014 Nov 5;6(261):261ra151-1.

[132] de Gooijer CJ, Borm FJ, Scherpereel A, Baas P. Immunotherapy in Malignant Pleural Mesothelioma. Front Oncol. 2020;10:187.

[133] Barsky AR, Cengel KA, Katz SI, Sterman DH, Simone CB. First-ever Abscopal Effect after Palliative Radiotherapy and Immuno-gene Therapy for Malignant Pleural Mesothelioma. Cureus. 2019 Feb 20;11(2):e4102.

[134] Kepp O, Galluzzi L, Martins I, Schlemmer F, Adjemian S, Michaud M, et al. Molecular determinants of immunogenic cell death elicited by anticancer chemotherapy. Cancer Metastasis Rev. Springer US; 2011 Mar;30(1):61-9.

[135] Galluzzi L, Kepp O, Kroemer G. Immunogenic cell death in radiation therapy. Oncoimmunology. 2014 Oct 27;2(10):e26536-3.

[136] Zelenay S, Reis e Sousa C. Adaptive immunity after cell death. Trends in Immunology. 2013 Jul;34(7):329-35.

[137] Dunn GP, Bruce AT, Ikeda H, Old LJ, Schreiber RD. Cancer immunoediting: from immunosurveillance to tumor escape. Nat Immunol. 2002;3(11):991-8.

[138] Schreiber RD, Old LJ, Smyth MJ. Cancer Immunoediting: Integrating Immunity's Roles in Cancer Suppression and Promotion. Science. American Association for the Advancement of Science; 2011 Mar 24;331(6024):1565-70.

[139] Abuodeh Y, Venkat P, Kim S. Systematic review of case reports on the abscopal effect. Current Problems in Cancer. Elsevier; 2016 Jan 1;40(1):25-37.

[140] Wu L, Wu MO, la Maza De L, Yun Z, Yu J, Zhao Y, et al. Targeting the inhibitory receptor CTLA-4 on T cells increased abscopal effects in murine mesothelioma model. Oncotarget. 2015 May 20;6(14):12468-80.

[141] Bolotin DA, Poslavsky S, Mitrophanov I, Shugay M, Mamedov IZ, Putintseva EV, et al. MiXCR: software for comprehensive adaptive immunity profiling. Nat Methods. Nature Publishing Group; 2015 May;12(5): 380-1.

[142] Mose LE, Selitsky SR, Bixby LM, Marron DL, Iglesia MD, Serody JS, et al. Assembly-based inference of B-cell receptor repertoires from short read RNA sequencing data with V'DJer. Bioinformatics. 2016 Dec 15;32(24):3729-34.

[143] Selitsky SR, Mose LE, Smith CC, Chai S, Hoadley KA, Dittmer DP, et al. Prognostic value of B cells in cutaneous melanoma. Genome Med. Genome Medicine; 2019 May 25;11(1):1-11.

[144] Victora GD, Nussenzweig MC. Germinal centers. Annu Rev Immunol. Annual Reviews; 2012;30(1):429-57.

[145] Traggiai E, Becker S, Subbarao K, Kolesnikova L, Uematsu Y, Gismondo MR, et al. An efficient method to make human monoclonal antibodies from memory B cells: potent neutralization of SARS coronavirus. Nat Med. 2004 Jul 11;10(8):871-5.

[146] Kwakkenbos MJ, van Helden PM, Beaumont T, Spits H. Stable long-term cultures of self-renewing B cells and their applications. Immunol Rev. 2016 Mar;270(1):65-77.

[147] Gilbert AE, Karagiannis P, Dodev T, Koers A, Lacy K, Josephs DH, et al. Monitoring the Systemic Human Memory B Cell Compartment of Melanoma Patients for Anti-Tumor IgG Antibodies. Lu S, editor. PLOS ONE [Internet]. Public Library of Science; 2011 Apr 29;6(4):e19330-15. Available from: http://dx.plos.org/10.1371/journal.pone.0019330

[148] Clargo AM, Hudson AR, Ndlovu W, Wootton RJ, Cremin LA, O'Dowd VL, et al. The rapid generation of recombinant functional monoclonal antibodies from individual, antigen-specific bone marrow-derived plasma cells isolated using a novel fluorescence-based method. MAbs. Taylor & Francis; 2014 Jan;6(1):143-59.

[149] Tickle S, Howells L, O'Dowd V, Starkie D, Whale K, Saunders M, et al. A fully automated primary screening system for the discovery of therapeutic antibodies directly from B cells. J Biomol Screen. SAGE PublicationsSage CA: Los Angeles, CA; 2015 Apr;20(4):492-7.

[150] Jin A, Ozawa T, Tajiri K, Obata T, Kondo S, Kinoshita K, et al. A rapid and

efficient single-cell manipulation method for screening antigen-specific antibody-secreting cells from human peripheral blood. Nat Med. Nature Publishing Group; 2009 Sep;15(9):1088-92.

[151] Corti D, Voss J, Gamblin SJ, Codoni G, Macagno A, Jarrossay D, et al. A neutralizing antibody selected from plasma cells that binds to group 1 and group 2 influenza A hemagglutinins. Science. 2011 Aug 12;333(6044):850-6.

[152] Walker LM, Phogat SK, Chan-Hui P-Y, Wagner D, Phung P, Goss JL, et al. Broad and potent neutralizing antibodies from an African donor reveal a new HIV-1 vaccine target. Science. 2009 Oct 9;326(5950):285-9.

[153] Dantas-Barbosa C, de Macedo Brigido M, Maranhao AQ. Antibody phage display libraries: contributions to oncology. Int J Mol Sci. Molecular Diversity Preservation International; 2012;13(5):5420-40.

[154] Alfaleh MA, Alsaab HO, Mahmoud AB, Alkayyal AA, Jones ML, Mahler SM, et al. Phage Display Derived Monoclonal Antibodies: From Bench to Bedside. Front Immunol. Frontiers; 2020;11:1986.

[155] Rothe A, Klimka A, Tur MK, Pfitzner T, Huhn M, Sasse S, et al. Construction of phage display libraries from reactive lymph nodes of breast carcinoma patients and selection for specifically binding human single chain Fv on cell lines. Int J Mol Med. Spandidos Publications; 2004 Oct;14(4):729-35.

[156] Rouet R, Jackson KJL, Langley DB, Christ D. Next-Generation Sequencing of Antibody Display Repertoires. Front Immunol. 2018 Feb 2;9:1315.

[157] An F, Drummond DC, Wilson S, Kirpotin DB, Nishimura SL, Broaddus VC, et al. Targeted drug delivery to mesothelioma cells using functionally selected internalizing human single-chain antibodies. Molecular Cancer Therapeutics. 2008 Mar 1;7(3):569-78.

[158] Lei X, Guan C-W, Song Y, Wang H. The multifaceted role of CD146/MCAM in the promotion of melanoma progression. Cancer Cell International. BioMed Central; 2015;15(1):3-11.

[159] de Kruijff I, Timmermans A, Bakker den M, Trapman-Jansen A, Foekens R, Meijer-Van Gelder M, et al. The Prevalence of CD146 Expression in Breast Cancer Subtypes and Its Relation to Outcome. Cancers. Multidisciplinary Digital Publishing Institute; 2018 May;10(5):134.

[160] Olajuyin AM, Olajuyin AK, Wang Z, Zhao X, Zhang X. CD146 T cells in lung cancer: its function, detection, and clinical implications as a biomarker and therapeutic target. Cancer Cell International. BioMed Central; 2019 Sep 25;:1-13.

[161] Bidlingmaier S, He J, Wang Y, An F, Feng J, Barbone D, et al. Identification of MCAM/CD146 as the target antigen of a human monoclonal antibody that recognizes both epithelioid and sarcomatoid types of mesothelioma. Cancer Res. American Association for Cancer Research; 2009 Feb 15;69(4):1570-7.

[162] Beije N, Kraan J, Bakker den MA, Maat APWM, van der Leest C, Cornelissen R, et al. Improved diagnosis and prognostication of patients with pleural malignant mesothelioma using biomarkers in pleural effusions and peripheral blood samples - a short report. Cell Oncol (Dordr). Springer Netherlands; 2017 Oct;40(5):511-9.

[163] Barbas CF, Kang AS, Lerner RA, Benkovic SJ. Assembly of combinatorial antibody libraries on phage surfaces: the

gene III site. Proc Natl Acad Sci USA. National Academy of Sciences; 1991 Sep 15;88(18):7978-82.

[164] Cai X, Garen A. Anti-melanoma antibodies from melanoma patients immunized with genetically modified autologous tumor cells: selection of specific antibodies from single-chain Fv fusion phage libraries. Proc Natl Acad Sci USA. 1995 Jul 3;92(14):6537-41.

[165] Wortzel RD, Urban JL, Philipps C, Fitch FW, Schreiber H. Independent immunodominant and immunorecessive tumor-specific antigens on a malignant tumor: antigenic dissection with cytolytic T cell clones. JI. 1983 May;130(5):2461-6.

Section 4

Rare Skin Diseases

Chapter 6

Therapy Development for Epidermolysis Bullosa

Josefina Piñón Hofbauer, Verena Wally, Christina Guttmann-Gruber, Iris Gratz and Ulrich Koller

Abstract

Although rare genodermatoses such as Epidermolysis bullosa have received more attention over the last years, no approved treatment options targeting causal mutations are currently available. Still, such diseases can be devastating, in some cases even associated with life-threatening secondary manifestations. Therefore, developing treatments that target disease-associated complications along with causal therapies remains the focus of current research efforts, in order to increase patient's quality of life and potentially their life expectancy. Epidermolysis bullosa is a genodermatosis that is caused by mutations in either one of 16 genes, predominantly encoding structural components of the skin and mucosal epithelia that are crucial to give these barrier organs physical and mechanical resilience to stress. The genetic heterogeneity of the disease is recapitulated in the high variability of phenotypic expressivity observed, ranging from minor and localized blistering to generalized erosions and wound chronification, rendering certain subtypes a systemic disease that is complicated by a plethora of secondary manifestations. During the last decades, several studies have focused on developing treatments for EB patients and significant progress has been made, as reflected by numerous publications, patents, and registered trials available. Overall, strategies range from causal to symptom-relieving approaches, and include gene, RNA and cell therapies, as well as drug developments based on biologics and small molecules. In this chapter, we highlight the most recent and promising approaches that are currently being investigated in order to provide effective treatments for patients with epidermolysis bullosa in the future.

Keywords: Epidermolysis bullosa, genodermatoses, gene therapy, drug development, wound healing, pruritus, fibrosis, squamous cell carcinoma

1. Introduction

Epidermolysis bullosa (EB) refers to a group of rare genodermatoses typically characterized by vulnerability of the skin to friction or trauma, leading to blistering and wounding to various extents, *i.e.* from localized and mild to generalized and severe, depending on the respective subtype of the disease. EB subtypes are classified according to the mutated gene, the resulting product of which is either functionally impaired or absent, and the level at which tissue cleavage occurs. While involvement in some subtypes are restricted to the skin, for others, extracutaneous organs (*i.e.* mucosa and eyes) may be involved, along with a multitude of secondary manifestations that significantly impair patients' life quality (QoL) and may even be life-threatening. Among these is the development of an aggressive form of cutaneous squamous cell carcinoma (cSCC) in patients with the severe dystrophic subtype of the disease [1–3].

Worldwide approximately 500,000 people suffer from EB, which can be classified into four major groups [1]. Mainly dominantly inherited mutations within genes encoding keratin 5, 14 and plectin lead to EB simplex (EBS), associated with intraepidermal blister formation (**Figure 1**). Mutations within genes, encoding laminin-332, type XVII collagen or integrin-α6β4, are the main causes of the junctional form of EB (JEB), characterized by tissue separation within the lamina lucida of the basement membrane zone (BMZ). The severe dystrophic variant of EB (DEB) is caused exclusively by mutations within the gene *COL7A1*, encoding type VII collagen, resulting in tissue separation within the sub-lamina densa (**Figure 1**). Kindler syndrome is caused by recessive mutations within the *KIND1* gene leading to a complete loss of encoded Kindlin-1 and blistering in multiple skin layers [1].

Despite advances in our understanding of the spectrum of pathologies associated with the different subtypes of EB, a systemic cure is still out of reach. However, the increasing number of trials that are being conducted reflects significant progress in clinical research, including strategies to correct and/or modulate the aberrant molecules and mechanisms underlying this devastating disease. [4–7] The remarkable differences between EB-types and numerous subtypes, renders the development of therapies a complex challenge, as both inter-subtype and inter-individual differences require the development of more personalized treatments.

Major complications in EB range from itch and pain, to a predisposition to wound chronification and tumor development, with molecular contributors deriving from various sources including different tissue-associated cell types, matrix components, as well as inflammatory events. The majority of these comorbidities, in and of themselves, are not unique to EB, so that the repurposing of clinically approved treatments against such symptoms represents an attractive path for a more rapid market approval of these compounds for EB. Furthermore, new

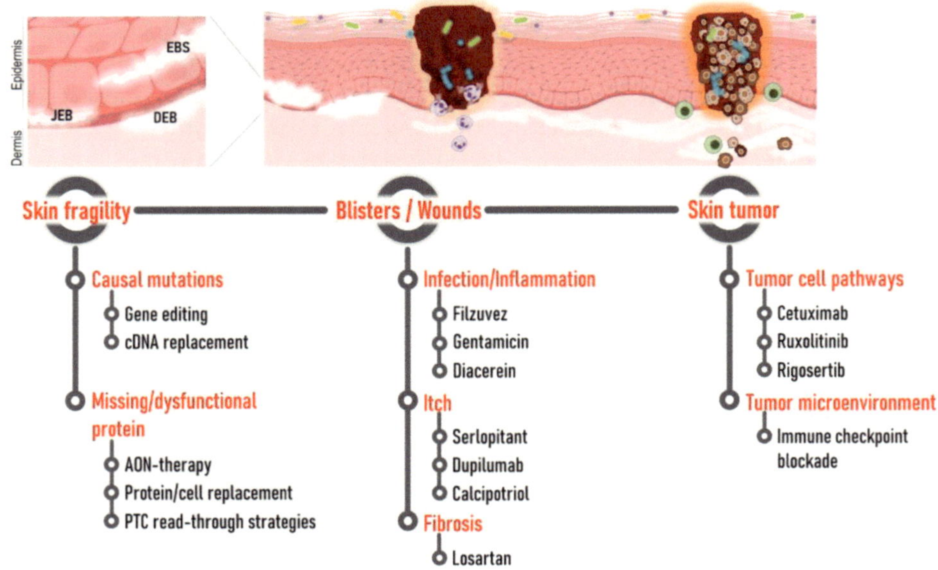

Figure 1.
Therapeutic targets in EB and strategies in development against them. EB is a rare hereditary skin fragility disorder characterized by blistering and wounding. In severe subtypes of the disease, wounds degenerate into tumors. The different therapeutic strategies to target important aspects of the disease are depicted.

evidence arising in the study of these common conditions can be leveraged to direct therapy development in EB. Nevertheless, rigorous evaluation for safety in this specific, vulnerable patient group is warranted for any candidate therapeutic. This is especially true for cancer therapies which are associated with significant cellular toxicity and often have the adverse effect of exacerbating the wound healing deficiencies associated with the disease.

2. Therapy development for EB

2.1 Causal therapies for epidermolysis bullosa

2.1.1 Gene replacement therapies for epidermolysis bullosa

The development of causal therapies has always been a main focus of EB research (**Table 1**).

Currently, gene replacement strategies that exploit viral vectors to introduce full-length wild type cDNA copies of the affected gene into the skin cells of patients [14], have advanced the furthest in clinical trials. However, this strategy relies on genomic integration of the transgene to achieve long-term restoration of gene

EB subtype	Therapeutic goal	Therapeutic strategy	Targeted gene/protein	Status	Ref
EB simplex	Causal therapy	Gene editing	*KRT5, KRT14*	pre-clinical	[8, 9]
		SMaRT	*KRT14, PLEC1*	pre-clinical	[10–13]
Junctional EB	Causal therapy	cDNA replacement	*LAMB3*	clinical	[14–17]
		Gene editing	*LAMB3*	pre-clinical	[18]
	Read-through therapy	PTC read-through	*LAMB3*	clinical	[7]
Recessive dystrophic EB	Causal therapy	cDNA replacement	*COL7A1*	clinical	[19–23]
		AON	*COL7A1*	pre-clinical	[24–27]
		Gene editing	*COL7A1*	pre-clinical	[24, 28–36]
		SMaRT	*COL7A1*	pre-clinical	[10, 37–40]
	Protein therapy	Protein replacement	Type VII vollagen	pre-clinical	[41]
	Cell therapy	Allogeneic fibroblast injection	Type VII collagen	clinical	[42]
	Read-through therapy	PTC read-through	*COL7A1*	clinical	[43]

Table 1.
Overview on causal therapies in epidermolysis bullosa and their current clinical status.

function, which bears a low risk of genomic toxicity due to insertional mutagenesis that can result in tumor development as shown for for X-linked severe combined immunodeficiency (X-SCID) [44]. However, no such deleterious events have been observed thus far for EB [14–17, 19]. In general, cutaneous gene therapies have the advantage that grafted skin areas are easy to monitor, with developing tumors easily detected and promptly excised. Until now, transplantation of genetically corrected skin grafts represents the most auspicious approach, due to the limited number of viral vectors suitable for *in vivo* targeting. Poor transcutaneous delivery of the vector and the size of the transgene represent further limitations [45, 46].

To date, the most successful application of gene replacement therapy has been achieved in junctional EB (JEB) patients carrying mutations in the *LAMB3* gene [14, 16, 17]. In all three cases, epidermal stem cells isolated from skin biopsies and expanded *in vitro*, were treated with a Moloney leukemia virus (MLV)-derived retroviral vector expressing the full-length cDNA of *LAMB3*. Treated cells were then expanded into epidermal sheets, which were transplanted back onto the patient. To this day, the first patient treated in 2006 still retains the transgenic epidermis, which at 6.5 years follow-up, appeared normal, blister-free, and showed accurate localized expression of laminin-332 within the skin, and no adverse effects reported thus far [15]. More recently, the same procedure was applied to treat an eight-year old JEB patient with life-threatening skin loss due to a bacterial infection. Over the course of successive treatments, up to ~80% of the patient's skin was surgically replaced by genetically corrected skin, demonstrating the life-saving potential of this therapeutic strategy for genodermatoses. Genetic analyses of the skin grafts clearly demonstrated that the transgenic epidermis was sustained by a defined number of epidermal stem cells with long-term regenerative potential [17].

Despite these successes, attempts to apply the same strategy in recessive dystrophic EB (RDEB) demonstrated no long-lasting effects. While long-term *COL7A1* expression could be attained following treatment, variable clinical outcomes were observed, with persistent type VII collagen expression detected in only two out of seven treated patients at two years post transplantation. [19, 20]

For most patients, improved wound healing and an accurate deposition of type VII collagen within the regenerated skin could be detected. However, expression of the transgene significantly decreased over time [19]. Possible reasons for this include the size of the *COL7A1* cDNA (~9 kb), the random nature of viral integrations, or post-transcriptional deregulation via aberrant splicing [21, 47]. In this respect, targeting *LAMB3* via a gene replacement therapy bears a big advantage over *COL7A1*, as the phenotype of JEB is associated with a significant depletion of epidermal stem cells [48]. Here, the YAP/TAZ mechano-sensing pathway plays a major role in sustaining holoclones downstream of Laminin-332 signaling. Holoclones represent stem cells with the greatest reproductive capacity and are essential for epidermal regeneration. Thus laminin-332 gene therapy likely rescues YAP activity, enabling the maintenance of the pool of epidermal stem cells [48]. Thus, while these clinical trials in JEB and DEB demonstrate the potential of gene replacement-based therapies in EB, they also reveal the varying therapeutic efficiencies that can be expected among the different EB types, potentially depending on the biology of the respective matrix protein affected.

In contrast to targeting patient keratinocytes, a combined gene and cell therapy approach using patient autologous fibroblasts was recently evaluated in a phase I, open-label, single-center clinical trial in four RDEB patients [22]. Based on previous preclinical data [23], patient fibroblasts were first modified *ex vivo* to carry a full-length codon-optimized *COL7A1* cDNA using a self-inactivating lentiviral vector. The gene-modified autologous fibroblasts were then injected intradermally back into the patients. The treatment was well-tolerated and no serious side effects were observed. Mean fluorescence intensity of type VII collagen staining in treated skin was 1.26-fold to 26.10-fold increased over non-injected skin, with enhanced expression sustained for up to 12 months in 2 out of the 4 patients [22]. This study demonstrated the potential of a combined gene & cell therapy approach for the treatment of RDEB, although more clinical data is required to evaluate the benefit for the patient.

2.1.2 Gene editing strategies for epidermolysis bullosa

Gene editing platforms based on programmable nucleases have advanced at a rapid pace, such that the correction of any gene is now, at least in theory, conceivable. At their core, designer nucleases consist of DNA endonucleases, such as zinc-finger nucleases (ZNF), transcription activator-like effector nucleases (TALEN) and clustered regularly interspaced short palindromic repeats (CRISPR) /CRISPR-associated protein 9 (Cas9), which are guided to specific DNA loci of interest, where they generate double-strand breaks (DSBs) and trigger the activation of DNA repair mechanisms [49, 50]. The most frequent repair pathway, termed non-homologous end joining pathway (NHEJ), relies on the introduction of small insertions and deletions (indels) at the DSB site [51], which can be leveraged for the inactivation of genes carrying dominant negative missense mutations [8, 52], or for the reframing of genes bearing pathogenic frameshift mutations [28, 29].

While not a genetic correction *per se*, gene disruption can be a suitable way of targeting dominant alleles via causing the coding sequence to run into a premature termination codon (PTC) during translation. Ribosomal stalling and activation of the nonsense-mediated mRNA decay pathway triggers the degradation of the edited mutant transcripts [53]. We have exploited this strategy to disrupt a dominant negative *KRT5* mutation whilst leaving the wild type allele intact [8]. This targeting strategy should be applicable to a broad number of EBS patients. Similarly, for DDEB, Shinkuma et al. applied an allele-specific gene disruption approach to target a dominant negative mutation within *COL7A1* [30].

The same strategy can also be used to reframe mutant mRNA and was recently shown by several groups to be a promising editing approach in RDEB [28, 29, 31, 32]. Leveraging recently developed algorithms to accurately predict end-joining (EJ) repair outcomes following CRISPR/Cas9-mediated cleavage, we were able to achieve significant restoration of *COL7A1* function after targeting a pathogenic frameshift mutation within exon 73 of *COL7A1* [29]. Sequence composition around the Cas9 binding site predicted a single adenine sense-strand insertion at the *COL7A1* target locus as the dominant EJ repair outcome, which would restore the reading frame of the message while introducing a single amino acid change in the protein. Indeed, we detected this precise nucleotide modification in 17% of all next generation sequencing (NGS)-analyzed *COL7A1* alleles, following a single RNP treatment. In all gene-edited cells analyzed, > 70% exhibited restored functional protein expression, underscoring the potential of end-joining based DNA repair strategies for restoring gene function in EB [29].

Of course, the holy grail of gene therapy has been to achieve a traceless repair of the disease-causing mutation. With current editing technologies, this is now attainable by invoking the high-fidelity homology directed repair (HDR) pathway. By providing an exogenous HDR donor sequence, which bears homology to the target region, the exchange of whole gene regions or individual nucleotides can be achieved [18, 24, 49, 50]. However, in comparison to EJ-based targeting strategies, gene editing efficiency is generally reduced, as homologous recombination is only active during the late S/G2 phase of the cell cycle [54]. Nevertheless, in EB, HDR-based gene repair strategies have been successfully applied to EBS [9] and

RDEB cells [24, 33, 35] *in vitro*. The focus of therapy development currently lies on improving safety and efficiency, which are both prerequisites for any future *in vivo* application of this strategy. Towards this end, to circumvent the known off-target activity of wild type *Streptococcus pyogenes* Cas9 (SpCas9), we utilized a mutant Cas9D10A nuclease, which predominantly induces single-strand nicks instead of double-strand breaks within the DNA [55, 56]. Indeed, we found that targeting of mutant *KRT14* or *COL7A1* alleles with two guided nickases in a double-nicking configuration was safer and more efficient than the use of wild type spCas9 [9, 24]. Additional efficiency can be gained by optimizing both, the format and the delivery of the gene-editing molecules. Currently, electroporation of *COL7A1*-specific RNPs together with single-stranded oligonucleotide HDR templates have resulted in the highest repair efficiencies [34].

The application of HDR-based approaches to the correction of patient-derived induced pluripotent stem cells (iPSCs) further increases the range of therapeutic options for patients, especially as the isolation of epidermal holoclones can be a limiting factor [14, 34]. Pre-clinical studies using corrected iPSCs, that were then differentiated into keratinocytes and fibroblasts, and used to generate three-dimensional skin equivalents (HSEs) on the backs of immunodeficient mice, showed normal type VII collagen expression and restored anchoring fibrils [34]. Alternative strategies, not based on homology-directed repair, comprise base editing, which has proven to be a suitable option for correcting pathogenic mutations in RDEB [36]. The most recent genome editing tool, prime editing, can be used to directly write new genetic information into a selected genomic locus using a Cas9 nickase fused to an engineered reverse transcriptase (RT) domain [57]. Via a prime editing guide RNA (pegRNA), which specifies the target site and represents the RT template encoding the desired edit, the prime editor is directed to the target locus. Here, the Cas9 nickase makes a single strand DNA break, that induces the hybridization of the nicked genomic strand to the complementary primer binding site (PBS) sequence, located within the pegRNA. A subsequent reverse transcription of the RT template, carrying the desired edit, followed by a cellular DNA repair mechanism lead to the insertion of the respective genetic modification at the target site [57]. Prime editing potentially improves safety, efficiency and applicability, and its application to EB will undoubtedly be confirmed in appropriate disease models in the near future.

2.1.3 RNA-based therapies for epidermolysis bullosa

A promising RNA-based strategy for the restoration of functional protein expression in EB is based on the use of antisense oligonucleotides (AON) for the specific knockdown of genes or their modification via splicing interference [58]. AONs are generally short fragments of modified DNA or RNA which, in the case of splicing modulation, hybridize to splicing elements (*e.g.* splice acceptor site or enhancers) within an in-frame target exon during pre-mRNA splicing, thereby masking it from the splicing machinery and resulting in its exclusion from the mature transcript. Thus, a truncated protein carrying an in-frame deletion of one or more exons is translated from the new transcript. In the last decade, AON-mediated splicing modulation has been successfully applied in DEB keratinocytes to skip in-frame *COL7A1* exon 70 [25], exon 73 [24, 26], exon 80 [26], and exon 105 [27] that carried dominant or recessive disease-causing mutations. The resulting proteins, though shorter, retained functionality. Indeed, *COL7A1* is amenable to AON-based exon skipping strategies because of the numerous short in-frame exons that encode its collagenous domains [24]. Beyond proof-of-concept, formulation of an exon 73-specific AON, named QR-313, within a carbomer-composed gel for topical treatment of wounds in DEB, led to enhanced type VII collagen levels in human RDEB skin [24], and is currently being evaluated for safety and efficacy in clinical trials (NCT03605069). However, not all exons are suitable targets for exon skipping. Furthermore, amino acid sequences potentially vital for protein function may be deleted. Thus, AON-based gene repair approaches need to be carefully evaluated for each targeted gene, exon and even mutation, prior to their clinical application [27].

Another RNA-based strategy for mRNA correction, namely RNA *trans*-splicing (also termed spliceosome-mediated RNA *trans*-splicing, SMaRT), has emerged as an attractive therapeutic option for the correction of EB-associated mutations on the RNA level [10–12]. Here, the endogenous splicing machinery is exploited to selectively exchange mutation-bearing regions of the target pre-mRNA, with the corresponding wild type sequence from an exogenously provided RNA *trans*-splicing molecule (RTM) [59]. The engineered RTM contains a binding domain to direct its hybridization to the target pre-mRNA, as well as splicing elements required for efficient splicing, in addition to the wild-type coding sequence to be restored [59]. This approach has been applied to accurately restore gene function in a variety of human genetic diseases, including hemophilia A [60], muscular dystrophy [61, 62] or Alzheimer's disease [63]. In EB, SMaRT-mediated RNA editing was first achieved for the *PLEC* gene [12], but has more recently, been used to correct the EB-associated genes *KRT14* [10, 11, 13] and *COL7A1* [37–40] *in vitro* and in pre-clinical animal models. However, while these studies indicated a potential clinical applicability of SMaRT technology in gene therapy for EB, the efficiency of this RNA-based method needs to be significantly improved if it is to move forward towards clinical translation.

2.1.4 Protein- and cell-based therapies for epidermolysis bullosa

Protein replacement strategies were recently applied in preclinical studies for RDEB. The local or intravenous injection of recombinant type VII collagen led to its homing to the dermal-epidermal junction and promoted wound healing [41]. Another therapeutic option for RDEB is the administration of type VII collagen-expressing allogeneic fibroblasts into healing RDEB wounds. Particularly when injected intradermally allogeneic fibroblast therapy resulted in a significant decrease in wound area when compared to standard of care after 2 and 12 weeks of treatment [42].

2.1.5 Read-through strategies for epidermolysis bullosa

Premature stop codon (PTC) read-through strategies rely on agents that allow for the incorporation of a random amino acid at the PTC position in the mRNA. Depending on the importance of the original amino acid to protein function, as well as impact of the introduced amino acid to *e.g.* protein folding, stability, and post-translational processing, PTC read-through therapies can result in the synthesis of a functional full-length protein. This strategy has been shown to be feasible in RDEB-derived cells [64, 65]. Cogan et al. treated RDEB keratinocyte cell lines and RDEB fibroblasts carrying PTC mutations, with the aminoglycosides geneticin, gentamicin and paromomycin. Full-length type VII collagen was accurately synthesized and secreted in a dose-dependent and sustained manner, highlighting the therapeutic potential of PTC read-through approaches for RDEB patients [65]. This resulted in a clinical trial to assess safety and efficacy of topical and intradermal gentamicin treatment in 5 RDEB patients with nonsense mutations application led to induced type VII collagen expression and anchoring fibril generation at the dermal-epidermal junction of treated skin areas, with improved wound closure and reduced blistering [43]. However, the toxicity associated with long-term aminoglycoside use currently hinders their widespread clinical application for these purposes. Alternatively, the FDA-approved anti-inflammatory drug amlexanox has been demonstrated to induce full-length collagen type VII expression *in vitro* in 8 out of 12 different RDEB PTC alleles tested. Furthermore, read-through synthesis correlated with the phosphorylation of the RNA helicase UPF-1, suggesting that inhibition of nonsense mediated decay of the PTC-containing mRNA contributed to its mechanism of action [64]. However, increased read-through translation alone is insufficient to achieve proper function, and additionally accurate deposition of the protein at the basement membrane zone likely needs to be confirmed for each PTC mutation. Similar to the mentioned RDEB studies, the aminoglycoside gentamicin was recently applied to JEB keratinocytes carrying various nonsense mutations within the *LAMB3* gene [66]. As a result, the authors achieved PTC read-through leading to the synthesis and secretion of the respective laminin chain protein as well as the restoration of laminin-332 assembly [66]. Nevertheless, future studies are required to address current issues concerning read-through-based approaches such as the toxicity and bioavailability of applied compounds and their interactions within treated cells and organisms.

In summary, numerous strategies to target the genetic cause of EB, as well as ameliorate disease-associated complications, are under intensive investigation. These act at various levels, from genes and gene products, to cellular pathways, tissue processes, and systemic events. While each strategy has distinct strengths and challenges, they all share the overarching aim of significatnly improving the QoL of patients (**Figure 2**).

2.1.6 Immunological aspects of causal therapy

Immunological tolerance to self-antigens result from central and peripheral tolerance mechanisms. Central tolerance in the thymus results in either negative selection of self-reactive T cells or development of self-specific suppressive regulatory T cells, both of which require expression and presentation of self-antigens to developing thymocytes. Additionally, various peripheral mechanisms of tolerance protect the body from deleterious reactions against self-tissues. These include anatomical sequestration of self-antigens, deletion of peripheral autoreactive lymphocytes, the development of functional unresponsiveness of lymphocytes (anergy) and action of regulatory T cells [67, 68].

A major risk in patients, especially those completely lacking expression of the affected protein, is that this protein is missing from the repertoire of self-antigens presented during central tolerance establishment. As the aim of causal therapies is to restore the missing protein or repair a defective (*e.g.* truncated) one, these include an inherent risk of inducing adverse immune reactivity against the restored wild type protein, at least parts of which would be recognized in patients as foreign. For these reasons, only patients with residual expression of the EB-associated protein have been included in gene therapy trials to date [14, 16, 17, 19]. Despite this, transient circulating antibodies reactive against the gene-correction product, and also tissue-bound antibodies deposited within the graft, were reported in some participants [19, 20]. However, these did not correlate with rejection of the graft. In addition, a phenomenon called epitope spreading could theoretically occur in patients that mount an immune reaction against the gene-correction product, leading to autoimmunity against the endogenous mutated/residual protein present throughout the body's epithelial tissues. This systemic immune reaction would likely manifest as blistering within the graft, as well as worsened blistering distal to the graft. Thus, monitoring immunological parameters (*e.g.* specific antibody formation) and diffuse new-onset blistering is warranted in study participants. While detailed immunological studies are still largely lacking, the results suggest ex vivo gene-replacement therapy to be a safe therapeutic approach in patients who lack pre-existing immune reactivity and express residual protein. However, future

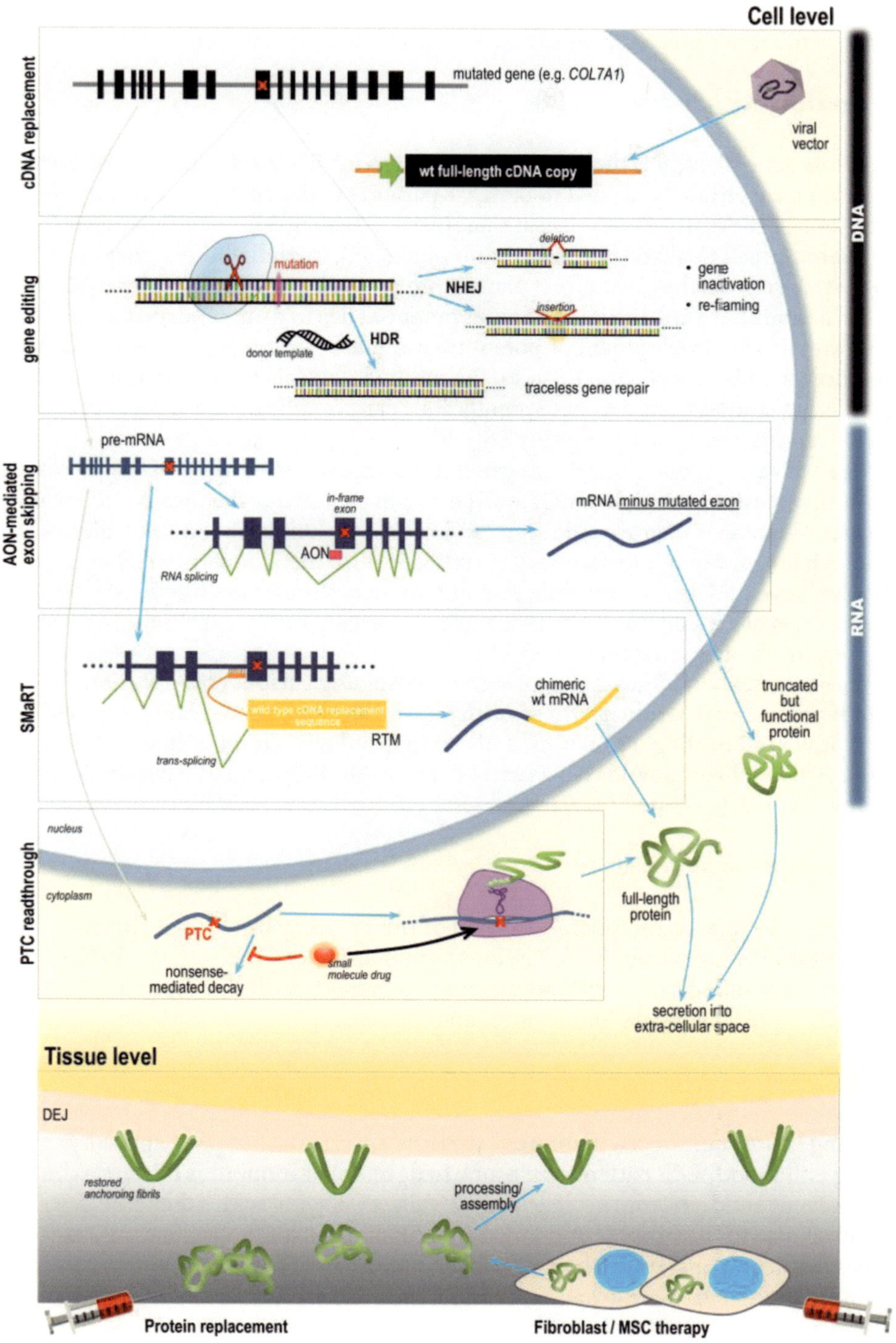

Figure 2.
Causal therapy options for epidermolysis bullosa. Current strategies targeting the genetic cause of EB can be designed to act either on DNA level (cDNA replacement, gene editing), RNA level (AON-mediated exon skipping, SMaRT), RNA/protein level (PTC readthrough) or tissue level (protein replacement fibroblast/ MSC therapy).

trials should aim to also include patients without any residual protein expression, who oftentimes display a more severe phenotype, and where there is likely no pre-existing tolerance to prevent adverse immune reactions against the gene-correction product. Towards this goal, further research is required to exploit peripheral immune tolerance mechanisms to control the response to neo-antigens in the skin.

2.2 Treating complications of EB

While gene therapy is the only curative option for EB, strategies to ameliorate symptoms are critically needed to increase patient's QoL and prevent severe complications of the disease until causal therapies are available for all EB patients. The number of preclinical and clinical studies published, including those currently registered, reflects the great effort placed into providing such. Strategies to identify suitable candidates are diverse, but great potential lies in drug repurposing, as this facilitates timely development of potent treatments by leveraging already existing pre-clinical and clinical data. Even so, the methodological challenges inherent to conducting studies in rare disease populations can complicate the clinical evaluation of repositioning such drugs for EB [69].

The active components of drugs generally comprise small molecules or biologics. While low molecular weight small molecules can be derived chemically and exhibit distinct advantages regarding delivery and route of administration, biologics, which are much larger, often interfere very specifically with distinct pathomechanisms and show overall less toxicity. Functionally, small molecules are frequently designed as inhibitors of *e.g.* enzymes, whereas biologics usually have a specific active function (*e.g.* antibodies, enzymes, nucleic acids).

In the context of EB several approaches addressing various complications have been reported, with the majority of primary outcomes measured being improvement of wound healing, reduction of blistering, and mitigation of itch. While some of the evaluated compounds have reached late stage clinical trials, first marketing approvals are still awaited [4–7, 69].

2.2.1 Reduction of blistering

Across the various EB types, blistering of the skin may be the first clinical manifestation of skin fragility following mechanical friction or trauma. While in some patients blisters heal without scarring, in patients suffering from more severe subtypes these degenerate into wounds and are accompanied by multiple comorbidities. Thus, preventing blistering or accelerating their resolution is a logical primary outcome measure for clinical trials due to its relevance to patients, at least in distinct patient cohorts [7]. Particularly in EBS, where patients only rarely develop wounds, reducing blister numbers will improve patients' QoL substantially. Especially during childhood, EBS patients are prone to developing numerous blisters, which may prevent children from *e.g.* learning to walk, or playing with other children. However, also for dystrophic and junctional EB clinical studies evaluating a treatment's impact on blister numbers have been published [7].

For EBS, uncovering the pathways and molecular mediators underscoring the pathogenic keratin biology in cells, proved instrumental to the development of a topical formulation of the drug diacerein, which has been shown in randomized controlled trials (RCTs) to significantly reduce blister numbers in comparison to patients who received placebo [70, 71]. Moreover, during the patient follow-up period when no treatment was applied, a delayed recurrence of blisters was observed, pointing towards a long-term stabilization of the skin. Diacerein is a small molecule that interferes with the expression and signaling of the pro-inflammatory cytokine IL-1ß at various levels. Upregulation of IL-1ß, triggered by the accumulation of mutated keratins, is characteristic for distinct subtypes of EBS. However, the reciprocal effect of IL-1ß to further induce the expression of mutant keratins was also observed in patient cells. Thus, interfering with this positive feedback loop proved beneficial to stabilizing the keratinocyte's intermediate filament network and consequently, also the patient's skin [72].

2.2.2 Wound healing

EB patients develop wounds throughout their lifetime, and their management and daily care routine represent a major burden that is accompanied by substantial discomfort. There is currently no standard treatment for the treatment of non-healing or severely infected wounds in EB. Defects in wound healing, associated with infections and persistent inflammation are presumed major drivers of wound chronification, which is a major risk factor for the development of particularly aggressive squamous cell carcinomas (SCC) [2, 3]. Thus, means to improve wound healing, and thereby prevent downstream complications that severely decrease QoL and that may even be life-threatening, are urgently needed. This is also reflected by the high number of clinical trials that primarily aim to improve wound healing, either by applying drugs that modulate wound healing associated pathways (*e.g.* modulation of inflammation), or, if feasible, by directly targeting the EB-causing gene products using drugs that induce read-through of PTCs.

Promising outcomes were recently reported from a trial using anti-inflammatory/immunomodulatory betulin-rich birch bark extract (Filzuvez, previously Oleogel S-10), wherein 41.3% of patients treated with Oleogel-S10 met the primary endpoint of target wound closure within 45 (± 7) days as compared to 28.9% of patients within the placebo arm. Furthermore, among the EB subtypes evaluated, patients with RDEB appeared to be particularly responsive to treatment (NCT03068780). In the context of wound healing, induction of PTC read-through as a means of triggering re-expression of genes harboring nonsense mutations, is particularly attractive in cases where the drugs being evaluated for these purposes have known antibacterial and anti-inflammatory activity. Particularly for junctional and dystrophic EB patients, clinical trials investigating the aminoglycoside antibiotic gentamicin are still ongoing [43, 73, 74] (NCT04140786, NCT03526159, NCT04644627, NCT03392909). Additionally for RDEB, the anti-inflammatory, anti-allergic immunomodulator Amlexanox, typically used against mouth ulcers, has emerged as a novel candidate in preclinical studies [64].

2.2.3 Pruritus

Pruritus is a particularly agonizing aspect associated with all subtypes of EB which not only impairs patients' QoL, but also leads to additional skin damage as it provokes scratching. Even though pruritus is not a life-threatening symptom *per se*, its overall influence on well-being is tremendous. In general, itch is a major problem associated with various diseases like atopic dermatitis, psoriasis, and nephrologic conditions. Yet, underlying molecular mechanisms are still not fully understood. Numerous inflammatory mediators have been associated with pathological itch, but despite pruritus being a severe clinical problem, effective treatments still represent an unmet medical need [75].

For patients with EB, a handful of studies targeting itch have been published, the most recent being a randomized-controlled trial (RCT) evaluating the neurokinin-1 receptor (NK1R) antagonist Serlopitant in patients with any EB subtype [76]. Serlopitant disrupts Substance P (SP) associated signaling by preventing its binding to NK1R. Expressed on multiple skin cell types, NK1R is thought to play a major role in the transmission of itch signals in the peripheral and central nervous systems [77]. In the RCT above, 14 EB patients received serlopitant or placebo over a period of 8 weeks, and reduction of pruritus was assessed using a numeric rating scale. Even though results were not statistically significant, patients who had received the investigational drug tended to achieve a ≥ 3 point reduction in itch compared to placebo, and a positive impact on QoL was reported by the patients. However, a larger clinical trial will be needed to provide clear evidence on the efficacy of serlopitant in reducing pruritus in patients with EB [76].

Another agent currently being evaluated against pruritus in patients with EB-pruriginosa is the anti-interleukin-4 receptor alpha (IL-4Rα) monoclonal antibody Dupilumab [78, 79]. Already indicated for atopic dermatitis, Dupilumab inhibits both IL-4 and IL-13 signaling and modulates Th2-mediated immune mechanisms. The promising outcome of both studies, which included a total of three patients, might provide a rationale for larger RCTs in the future that extend to other subtypes of EB.

Interestingly, in a single-patient observational study aimed primarily at investigating the wound healing benefits of a low-dose topical calcipotriol ointment in DEB, a significant reduction of itch was reported as a highly patient-relevant outcome. Calcipotriol is an analogue of the active form of vitamin D3, an important skin homeostasis factor with roles in cell proliferation, differentiation, antimicrobial defense, and immune modulation. Calcipotriol has proven anti-proliferative effects in keratinocytes, which is leveraged for the treatment of plaque psoriasis. For this reason, we investigated a lower concentration with respect to antimicrobial peptide induction in DEB keratinocytes. In addition to the complete closure of a chronic wound within two weeks of treatment, we observed significant improvement in the diversity of the skin microbiota on the treated skin area, with complete clearance of *Staphylococcus aureus* by the end of the treatment [80]. The low dose ointment was evaluated in a small double-blind, placebo-controlled phase II clinical trial (EudraCT: 2016–001967-35), where a significant and steady reduction in pruritus was observed with calcipotriol treatment compared to placebo [81]. These results support conducting a follow-up trial to investigate its impact on itch in patients with EB, particularly given calcipotriol's reported anti-neoplastic effects.

2.2.4 Fibrosis

Repeated cycles of injury and subsequent persistent inflammation trigger a cascade of events leading to progressive fibrosis, followed by tissue stiffening and increased risk of tumor development in patients with dystrophic EB. Additionally, fibrotic webbing at limb extremities post-wounding ultimately leads to fusion of fingers and toes (called mitten deformities), severely limiting their use. Thus, strategies to support a normal course of wound healing are investigated to avoid or minimize deviations from deposition of a normal skin matrix [82]. A key player in EB-associated fibrosis is TGF-ß, a pro-inflammatory cytokine whose pleiotropic effects are highly context-dependent, and which has been shown to be constitutively expressed in RDEB-skin [83, 84]. While TGF-ß1 promotes wound healing under normal conditions, excessive TGF-ß1 signaling leads to abnormal ECM deposition and scar formation, as confirmed in a type VII collagen hypomorphic mouse model [85, 86]. Thus, modulating the expression of TGF-ß1 was hypothesized to be beneficial in reducing fibrosis. In this context, losartan, an angiotensin II antagonist with anti-fibrotic effects, has been evaluated in preclinical studies, where Nystrom *et al* achieved a significant reduction in fibrosis in collagen VII hypomorphic mice. This approach led to reduced TGF-ß signaling, normalized skin extracellular matrix composition, and delayed progression of mitten deformities [83]. Based on these results, a phase I/II clinical trial to evaluate the safety, tolerability and efficacy of losartan in children and adolescents with RDEB is currently underway (Eudra-CT: 2015–003670-32).

In a drug repurposing approach, endoglin (CD105), a type III co-receptor for TGF-1, and raloxifene, an estrogen receptor modulator, were tested in a pre-clinical setting for their potential to attenuate RDEB-associated fibrosis. Indeed, both drugs were shown to modulate profibrotic events, rendering them potential candidates for repositioning both compounds for the treatment of patients with EB [86].

2.3 EB-associated squamous cell carcinoma

Cutaneous tumors are a life-threatening complication that arise especially in patients with RDEB. Owing to the repeated cycles of wounding, infection and inflammation, RDEB patients are at especially high risk of developing aggressive squamous cell carcinoma (RDEB-SCC) with high risk-features. The sites of tumor occurrence are predominantly at sites of chronic and long-term wounds [87], especially on the extremities [88], indicating that tumorigenesis is related to the pathology of RDEB. The SCCs tend to arise in early adulthood, with a reported median age of 29 years at time of diagnosis, although the youngest case reported was in a 6-year old patient [89]. In comparison to the general population, RDEB patients have an estimated 70-fold higher risk of developing SCC [90], with cumulative risk rising from 7.5% at age 20 years, to 67.8% at age 35 years, to 90.1% by age 55 [2]. Despite aggressive therapy with multiple treatment modalities, median survival time from time of first diagnosis is 4–5 years [89], making RDEB-SCC the primary cause of premature death in these patients. The first choice of treatment still consists of wide local excision of the tumor, and even amputation of the extremity is sometimes necessary. Radiotherapy and conventional chemotherapeutic approaches have been mostly used palliatively in EB SCC and considering their strong adverse effects (*e.g.* desquamation of the skin upon radiotherapy) should be used carefully when applied to this vulnerable patient group [91].

Genomic analyses combined with transcriptomic profiling of tumors highlight cell endogenous mutagenic processes mediated by APOBEC enzymes, which are associated with an innate defense mechanism against ongoing microbial infection, as a major driver of carcinogenesis in RDEB. These observations indicate that effective wound management, which includes an antimicrobial component, could potentially lower cancer risk in these patients. Genetically, RDEB-SCC closely resembles ultraviolet (UV) light-induced SCC and SCC of the head and neck (HN-SCC), with driver mutations in known cancer-associated genes such as *CASP8, NOTCH1, TP53, FAT1, CDKN2A, HRAS, ARID2, and KMT2B* frequently observed [92]. While these similarities suggest that therapies proven to be efficacious in other SCCs would also be effective in RDEB SCC, careful consideration of the background pathology of EB is needed. The significant overlap in cellular processes associated with wound healing and tumor development (*e.g.* proliferation, migration, vascularisation/angiogenesis, matrix remodeling) dictates that a delicate balance needs to established wherein tumor inhibition is not interfering with wound healing, especially when long-term treatment is considered.

2.3.1 EGFR inhibition

Cetuximab, a monoclonal antibody targeting the extracellular domain of epidermal growth factor receptor (EGFR), has been used for therapy against both HN-SCC, as well as advanced unresectable cutaneous UV-SCC [93, 94]. This agent inhibits tumor cell proliferation by blocking receptor tyrosine kinase activity upstream of known survival-, growth-, and migration- signaling cascades mediated by *PI3K/AKT*, *RAS/MAPK*, and *JAK/STAT* [95, 96]. Cetuximab shows significant efficacy against EGFR-positive, wild type RAS tumors, while those bearing RAS mutations are resistant to treatment [97]. EB-associated SCCs frequently express EGFR, but with noticeable differences in expression level which could impact responsiveness to treatment [98]. To date, only a handful of cases have reported the use of cetuximab in EB patients with advanced cutaneous SCC, with limited beneficial effects on survival [88, 94, 98–100]. Progression-free survival in seven patients reported in the literature ranged from three weeks to nine months. Better outcomes have been observed when cetuximab was given as a first line treatment suggesting that treatment might be more efficacious when administered early. Of note, wound healing deficits and worsening of skin lesions, which negatively impact patient's QoL, were noted in three patients. For one patient, the negative effects on patient wound healing led to a dose reduction of cetuximab and subsequent tumor recurrence soon after [98]. This negative impact of cetuximab in RDEB is likely associated with the important roles of the aforementioned downstream signaling cascades in wound healing processes and exemplifies the challenge of treating tumors in the background of EB. Thus, more targeted strategies, aimed at inhibition of tumor-essential pathways downstream of EGFR are already being investigated and are expected to minimize such adverse effects.

2.3.2 JAK1/2 inhibition

The Janus kinase/signal transducers and activators of transcription (JAK/STAT) pathway mediates cellular responses to a variety of cytokines and growth factors, including IL-6 and EGF, downstream of these ligands binding their cognate receptors. These responses include proliferation, differentiation, migration, survival, and apoptosis, and are dependent on cell- and tissue-type, as well as the context of the signal [101]. In this respect JAK/STAT plays important roles in developmental and homeostatic processes, and is also aberrantly active in numerous cancers, including HN-SCC [102]. Increased levels of phosphorylated STAT3, a downstream effector of JAK, were observed in RDEB-SCC cells over normal keratinocytes, providing rationale for evaluating the effect of the JAK1/2 inhibitor ruxolitinib in a murine xenograft model of human RDEB-SCC [103]. In this preclinical study, ruxolitinib effectively reduced tumor mass, when administered either orally or topically onto tumors, because reduced STAT3 signaling led to decreased cell proliferation. These observations argue that ruxolitinib may be a promising anticancer drug for RDEB-SCC. When ruxolitinib was used with the aim to counteract the fibrotic processes in the skin of type VII collagen hypomorphic mice, a reduction of phosphorylated STAT3 in fibroblasts and SCC *in vitro*, but only limited therapeutic benefit against fibrosis-driven mitten deformities in type VII collagen hypomorphic mice was observed [104]. Additionally, the drug was not well tolerated by the mice and, even more importantly, treatment delayed wound healing, highlighting that caution and rigorous evaluation is warranted before its clinical application in patients.

2.3.3 Polo-like kinase 1 inhibition

Due to the aggressive and metastasising nature of RDEB-SCC, which is atypical of UV-induced cutaneous SCCs that arise in the general population, gene expression assays were performed to identify differentially regulated genes that might account for this difference in tumor behavior. Among the handful of genes identified was polo-like kinase 1 (PLK1) [105], a serine/threonine protein kinase which was over-expressed in a number of different tumors [106]. Blocking PLK1 leads to mitotic arrest, inhibition of cell proliferation and apoptosis. Notably, cells were more sensitive to PLK1 inhibition when p53 was defective [107]. *TP53* is frequently mutated in RDEB-SCC [92] highlighting PLK1-inhibition as a potential strategy to selectively target tumor cells over normal cells which exhibit normal p53 function. Several small molecules are under investigation for their ability to target PLK1 signaling in cancer, and results from these studies can be leveraged to facilitate the evaluation of these agents also for clinical use in RDEB patients. A study by Atansova et al., identified rigosertib (or ON-01910) among six different small-molecule inhibitors of PLK1 as a strong and selective inducer of apoptosis in RDEB-SCC cells. Its pre-clinical evaluation in a murine xenograft model demonstrated inhibition of tumor growth without obvious toxicity, laying the path for a multi-center phase II clinical trial in RDEB patients with late stage, metastatic, and/or unresectable SCC. [64] (NCT03786237).

2.3.4 Immune checkpoint blocking

Immune checkpoints are molecules that are either able to turn on (co-stimulatory molecules) or turn off (inhibitory molecules) immune signaling, generally referring to the activation of responses in T cells. Tumors have developed mechanisms to exploit these immune checkpoint molecules in order to evade immune surveillance and escape clearance by *e.g.* cytotoxic T cells [108]. Such immune checkpoint molecules include CTLA-4 (cytotoxic T-lymphocyte-associated protein 4) and PD-1 (programmed death-1). The latter is predominantly expressed on T cells, and by binding to its ligands PD-L1 and PD-L2 expressed on tumor cells, induces a negative signal that leads to effector T cell suppression [109]. Blocking these interactions using specific antibodies leads to reactivation of the immune system and improvement of anti-tumor immune responses. Remarkable anti-tumor effects were achieved with an antibody targeting CTLA-4 (ipilimumab), increasing median overall survival in metastatic melanoma patients [109]. Even better outcomes in survival rate have been observed with pembrolizumab, an anti-PD1 receptor antibody [110]. Furthermore, beneficial evidence in clinical trials using anti-PD1 treatment in advanced HN-SCC [111], and also locally advanced/metastatic SCC [112] support PD-1 blocking as well in RDEB SCC. In this respect, 2 reports can be found in the literature describing the use of anti-PD1 blocking antibodies in RDEB-SCC patients. The first case described the use of pembrolizumab (PD-1 antibody) as second line therapy after cetuximab treatment. Pembrolizumab was partly combined with other therapeutic approaches including intralesional administration of talimogene laherparepvec (T-Vec; oncolytic virus) into metastatic tumors, radiotherapy and anti-EGFR monoclonal antibody (panitumumab). Wound healing was not impaired during the late stage of the disease. The patient died due to tumor progression 18 months after starting pembrolizumab treatment [100]. Most recently, Khaddour et al. report on an RDEB patient with metastatic SCC who was treated with cemiplimab (monoclonal anti-PD1) every 3 weeks in combination with radiotherapy. During the 14-month follow-up the patient showed a durable response with no signs of immune-related adverse events [113]. These observations support conducting controlled clinical trials to assess the efficacy of PD-1 blockade in this patient group. Noteworthy, another anti-PD1 antibody (nivolumab) is currently under evaluation in a multi-centre phase II clinical trial for the palliative treatment of EB patients with advanced or metastatic squamous cell carcinomas (EudraCT: 2016–002811-16) [6].

3. Conclusions

In the last decade, the number of clinical trials registered for the evaluation of therapies against various primary and secondary pathologies associated with the various forms of EB has risen dramatically (>70 clinical trials; clinicaltrials.

gov). They reflect the progress in the optimization of previous gene therapeutic approaches, discovery and advancement of novel gene editing technologies, and the increase in our understanding of the molecular and cellular mechanisms underpinning the nature of these EB-related complications. Drug repositioning has largely been prioritized, as leveraging the existing pharmacological and safety data represents the fastest and most economical route to clinical trials, and when successful, to marketing approval for EB. To further support the development of new therapy options for rare diseases like EB, several programs, like the orphan designation program by the European Medicines Agency (EMA) have been launched.

This is good news for patients, but also creates challenges for the recruitment of sufficient participants to the various trials, due to the rarity of the disease, strict inclusion criteria, and the disinclination of patients to participate. This heightens the risk of recruitment failure and the inability to meet statistical endpoints, resulting in extended trials that come at increased costs. Surmounting these challenges will require close collaboration within the entire EB community, to establish an international patient registry, incentivize patient participation, address logistical and regulatory aspects of multi-center trials, and allow for new outcome measures and the development of statistical methods for small cohorts. In parallel, applying current state-of-the-art methods that maximize acquisition of multi-modal data from patient samples, alongside the continuing advances in artificial intelligence, will further support the development of new therapies at various levels, starting from *in silico* drug discovery to establishing new means for measuring patient-relevant trial outcomes.

Acknowledgements

The authors would like to thank DEBRA Austria for their continued support and funding of our work. This work is generated within the ERN skin.

Conflict of interest

The authors declare no conflict of interest.

Author details

Josefina Piñón Hofbauer[1†], Verena Wally[1*†], Christina Guttmann-Gruber[1†], Iris Gratz[1,2†] and Ulrich Koller[1†]

1 Department of Dermatology and Allergology, EB House Austria, Research Program for Molecular Therapy of Genodermatoses, University Hospital of the Paracelsus Medical University Salzburg, Salzburg, Austria

2 Department of Biosciences, University of Salzburg, Salzburg, Austria

*Address all correspondence to: v.wally@salk.at

† All authors contributed equally.

References

[1] Has C, Bauer JW, Bodemer C, Bolling MC, Bruckner-Tuderman L, Diem A, et al. Consensus reclassification of inherited epidermolysis bullosa and other disorders with skin fragility. Br J Dermatol. 2020;183(4):614-627.

[2] Fine JD, Johnson LB, Weiner M, Li KP, Suchindran C. Epidermolysis bullosa and the risk of life-threatening cancers: the National EB Registry experience, 1986-2006. J Am Acad Dermatol. 2009;60(2):203-211.

[3] Condorelli AG, Dellambra E, Logli E, Zambruno G, Castiglia D. Epidermolysis Bullosa-Associated Squamous Cell Carcinoma: From Pathogenesis to Therapeutic Perspectives. Int J Mol Sci. 2019;20(22).

[4] Has C, South A, Uitto J. Molecular Therapeutics in Development for Epidermolysis Bullosa: Update 2020. Mol Diagn Ther. 2020;24(3):299-309.

[5] Uitto J. Toward treatment and cure of epidermolysis bullosa. Proc Natl Acad Sci U S A. 2019.

[6] Prodinger C, Reichelt J, Bauer JW, Laimer M. Epidermolysis bullosa: Advances in research and treatment. Exp Dermatol. 2019;28(10):1176-1189.

[7] Wally V, Reisenberger M, Kitzmuller S, Laimer M. Small molecule drug development for rare genodermatoses - evaluation of the current status in epidermolysis bullosa. Orphanet J Rare Dis. 2020;15(1):292.

[8] Aushev M, Koller U, Mussolino C, Cathomen T, Reichelt J. Traceless Targeting and Isolation of Gene-Edited Immortalized Keratinocytes from Epidermolysis Bullosa Simplex Patients. Mol Ther Methods Clin Dev. 2017;6: 112-123.

[9] Kocher T, Peking P, Klausegger A, Murauer EM, Hofbauer JP, Wally V, et al. Cut and Paste: Efficient Homology-Directed Repair of a Dominant Negative KRT14 Mutation via CRISPR/Cas9 Nickases. Mol Ther. 2017;25(11): 2585-2598.

[10] Peking P, Breitenbach JS, Ablinger M, Muss WH, Poetschke FJ, Kocher T, et al. An ex vivo RNA trans-splicing strategy to correct human generalized severe epidermolysis bullosa simplex. Br J Dermatol. 2019;180(1):141-148.

[11] Wally V, Brunner M, Lettner T, Wagner M, Koller U, Trost A, et al. K14 mRNA reprogramming for dominant epidermolysis bullosa simplex. Hum Mol Genet. 2010;19(23):4715-4725.

[12] Wally V, Klausegger A, Koller U, Lochmuller H, Krause S, Wiche G, et al. 5′ trans-splicing repair of the PLEC1 gene. J Invest Dermatol. 2008;128(3):568-574.

[13] Liemberger B, Pinon Hofbauer J, Wally V, Arzt C, Hainzl S, Kocher T, et al. RNA Trans-Splicing Modulation via Antisense Molecule Interference. Int J Mol Sci. 2018;19(3).

[14] Mavilio F, Pellegrini G, Ferrari S, Di Nunzio F, Di Iorio E, Recchia A, et al. Correction of junctional epidermolysis bullosa by transplantation of genetically modified epidermal stem cells. Nat Med. 2006;12(12):1397-1402.

[15] De Rosa L, Carulli S, Cocchiarella F, Quaglino D, Enzo E, Franchini E, et al. Long-term stability and safety of transgenic cultured epidermal stem cells in gene therapy of junctional epidermolysis bullosa. Stem Cell Reports. 2014;2(1):1-8.

[16] Bauer JW, Koller J, Murauer EM, De Rosa L, Enzo E, Carulli S, et al. Closure of a Large Chronic Wound through Transplantation of Gene-Corrected Epidermal Stem Cells. J Invest Dermatol. 2017;137(3):778-781.

[17] Hirsch T, Rothoeft T, Teig N, Bauer JW, Pellegrini G, De Rosa L, et al. Regeneration of the entire human epidermis using transgenic stem cells. Nature. 2017;551(7680):327-332.

[18] Benati D, Miselli F, Cocchiarella F, Patrizi C, Carretero M, Baldassarri S, et al. CRISPR/Cas9-Mediated In Situ Correction of LAMB3 Gene in Keratinocytes Derived from a Junctional Epidermolysis Bullosa Patient. Mol. Ther. 2018, 26, 2592-2603.

[19] Siprashvili Z, Nguyen NT, Gorell ES, Loutit K, Khuu P, Furukawa LK, et al. Safety and Wound Outcomes Following Genetically Corrected Autologous Epidermal Grafts in Patients With Recessive Dystrophic Epidermolysis Bullosa. JAMA. 2016;316(17):1808-17.

[20] Eichstadt S, Barriga M, Ponakala A, Teng C, Nguyen NT, Siprashvili Z, et al. Phase 1/2a clinical trial of gene-corrected autologous cell therapy for recessive dystrophic epidermolysis bullosa. JCI Insight. 2019;4(19).

[21] Titeux M, Pendaries V, Hovnanian A. Gene therapy for recessive dystrophic epidermolysis bullosa. Dermatol Clin. 2010;28(2):361-366, xii.

[22] Lwin SM, Syed F, Di WL, Kadiyirire T, Liu L, Guy A, et al. Safety and early efficacy outcomes for lentiviral fibroblast gene therapy in recessive dystrophic epidermolysis bullosa. JCI Insight. 2019;4(11).

[23] Georgiadis C, Syed F, Petrova A, Abdul-Wahab A, Lwin SM, Farzaneh F, et al. Lentiviral Engineered Fibroblasts Expressing Codon-Optimized COL7A1 Restore Anchoring Fibrils in RDEB. J Invest Dermatol. 2016;136(1):284-292.

[24] Kocher T, Wagner RN, Klausegger A, Guttmann-Gruber C, Hainzl S, Bauer JW, et al. Improved Double-Nicking Strategies for COL7A1-Editing by Homologous Recombination. Mol Ther Nucleic Acids. 2019;18:496-507.

[25] Goto M, Sawamura D, Nishie W, Sakai K, McMillan JR, Akiyama M, et al. Targeted skipping of a single exon harboring a premature termination codon mutation: implications and potential for gene correction therapy for selective dystrophic epidermolysis bullosa patients. J Invest Dermatol. 2006;126(12):2614-2620.

[26] Turczynski S, Titeux M, Pironon N, Hovnanian A. Antisense-mediated exon skipping to reframe transcripts. Methods Mol Biol. 2012;867:221-238.

[27] Bremer J, Bornert C, Nystrom A, Gostynski A, Jonkman MF, Aartsma-Rus A, et al. Antisense Oligonucleotide-mediated Exon Skipping as a Systemic Therapeutic Approach for Recessive Dystrophic Epidermolysis Bullosa. Mol Ther Nucleic Acids. 2016;5(10):e379.

[28] Takashima S, Shinkuma S, Fujita Y, Nomura T, Ujiie H, Natsuga K, et al. Efficient Gene Reframing Therapy for Recessive Dystrophic Epidermolysis Bullosa with CRISPR/Cas9. J Invest Dermatol. 2019;139(8):1711-1721 e4.

[29] Kocher T, March OP, Bischof J, Liemberger B, Hainzl S, Klausegger A, et al. Predictable CRISPR/Cas9-Mediated COL7A1 Reframing for Dystrophic Epidermolysis Bullosa. J Invest Dermatol. 2020;140(10):1985-1993 e5.

[30] Shinkuma S, Guo Z, Christiano AM. Site-specific genome editing for correction of induced pluripotent stem cells derived from dominant dystrophic epidermolysis bullosa. Proc Natl Acad Sci U S A. 2016;113(20):5676-5681.

[31] Chamorro C, Mencia A, Almarza D, Duarte B, Buning H, Sallach J, et al. Gene Editing for the Efficient Correction of a Recurrent COL7A1 Mutation in Recessive Dystrophic Epidermolysis Bullosa Keratinocytes. Mol Ther Nucleic Acids. 2016;5:e307.

[32] Mencia A, Chamorro C, Bonafont J, Duarte B, Holguin A, Illera N, et al. Deletion of a Pathogenic Mutation-Containing Exon of COL7A1 Allows Clonal Gene Editing Correction of RDEB Patient Epidermal Stem Cells. Mol Ther Nucleic Acids. 2018;11:68-78.

[33] Hainzl S, Peking P, Kocher T, Murauer EM, Larcher F, Del Rio M, et al. COL7A1 Editing via CRISPR/Cas9 in Recessive Dystrophic Epidermolysis Bullosa. Mol Ther. 2017;25(11):2573-2584.

[34] Jackow J, Guo Z, Hansen C, Abaci HE, Doucet YS, Shin JU, et al. CRISPR/Cas9-based targeted genome editing for correction of recessive dystrophic epidermolysis bullosa using iPS cells. Proc Natl Acad Sci U S A. 2019.

[35] Izmiryan A, Ganier C, Bovolenta M, Schmitt A, Mavilio F, Hovnanian A. Ex Vivo COL7A1 Correction for Recessive Dystrophic Epidermolysis Bullosa Using CRISPR/Cas9 and Homology-Directed Repair. Mol Ther Nucleic Acids. 2018;12: 554-567.

[36] Osborn MJ, Newby GA, McElroy AN, Knipping F, Nielsen SC, Riddle MJ, et al. Base Editor Correction of COL7A1 in Recessive Dystrophic Epidermolysis Bullosa Patient-Derived Fibroblasts and iPSCs. J Invest Dermatol. 2020;140(2):338-347 e5.

[37] Peking P, Koller U, Duarte B, Murillas R, Wolf S, Maetzig T, et al. An RNA-targeted therapy for dystrophic epidermolysis bullosa. Nucleic Acids Res. 2017;45(17):10259-10269.

[38] Murauer EM, Gache Y, Gratz IK, Klausegger A, Muss W, Gruber C, et al. Functional correction of type VII collagen expression in dystrophic epidermolysis bullosa. J Invest Dermatol. 2011;131(1): 74-83.

[39] Murauer EM, Koller U, Hainzl S, Wally V, Bauer JW. A reporter-based screen to identify potent 3′ trans-splicing molecules for endogenous RNA repair. Hum Gene Ther Methods. 2013;24(1): 19-27.

[40] Tockner B, Kocher T, Hainzl S, Reichelt J, Bauer JW, Koller U, et al. Construction and validation of an RNA trans-splicing molecule suitable to repair a large number of COL7A1 mutations. Gene Ther. 2016;23(11):775-784.

[41] Woodley DT, Wang X, Amir M, Hwang B, Remington J, Hou Y, et al. Intravenously injected recombinant human type VII collagen homes to skin wounds and restores skin integrity of dystrophic epidermolysis bullosa. J Invest Dermatol. 2013;133(7):1910-1913.

[42] Moravvej H, Abdollahimajd F, Naseh MH, Piravar Z, Abolhasani E, Mozafari N, et al. Cultured allogeneic fibroblast injection vs. fibroblasts cultured on amniotic membrane scaffold for dystrophic epidermolysis bullosa treatment. Br J Dermatol. 2018;179(1):72-79.

[43] Woodley DT, Cogan J, Hou Y, Lyu C, Marinkovich MP, Keene D, et al. Gentamicin induces functional type VII collagen in recessive dystrophic epidermolysis bullosa patients. J Clin Invest. 2017;127(8):3028-3038.

[44] Hacein-Bey-Abina S, Von Kalle C, Schmidt M, McCormack MP, Wulffraat N, Leboulch P, et al. LMO2-associated clonal T cell proliferation in two patients after gene therapy for SCID-X1. Science. 2003;302(5644): 415-419.

[45] Chamcheu JC, Wood GS, Siddiqui IA, Syed DN, Adhami VM, Teng JM, et al. Progress towards genetic and pharmacological therapies for keratin genodermatoses: current perspective and future promise. Exp Dermatol. 2012;21(7):481-489.

[46] Sallach J, Di Pasquale G, Larcher F, Niehoff N, Rubsam M, Huber A, et al.

Tropism-modified AAV vectors overcome barriers to successful cutaneous therapy. Mol Ther. 2014;22(5):929-939.

[47] Montini E, Cesana D, Schmidt M, Sanvito F, Bartholomae CC, Ranzani M, et al. The genotoxic potential of retroviral vectors is strongly modulated by vector design and integration site selection in a mouse model of HSC gene therapy. J Clin Invest. 2009;119(4):964-975.

[48] De Rosa, L., Secone Seconetti, A., De Santis, G., Pellacani, G., Hirsch, T., Rothoeft, T., et al. Laminin 332-Dependent YAP Dysregulation Depletes Epidermal Stem Cells in Junctional Epidermolysis Bullosa. Cell reports 2019;27, 2036-2049.

[49] March OP, Kocher T, Koller U. Context-Dependent Strategies for Enhanced Genome Editing of Genodermatoses. Cells. 2020;9(1).

[50] Kocher T, Koller U. Advances in Gene Editing Strategies for Epidermolysis Bullosa. Prog Mol Biol Transl Sci. 2021; doi:10.1016/bs.pmbts.2020.12.007.

[51] Brinkman EK, Chen T, de Haas M, Holland HA, Akhtar W, van Steensel B. Kinetics and Fidelity of the Repair of Cas9-Induced Double-Strand DNA Breaks. Mol Cell. 2018;70(5):801-813 e6.

[52] March OP, Lettner T, Klausegger A, Ablinger M, Kocher T, Hainzl S, et al. Gene Editing-Mediated Disruption of Epidermolytic Ichthyosis-Associated KRT10 Alleles Restores Filament Stability in Keratinocytes. J Invest Dermatol. 2019;139(8):1699-1710 e6.

[53] Santiago Y, Chan E, Liu PQ, Orlando S, Zhang L, Urnov FD, et al. Targeted gene knockout in mammalian cells by using engineered zinc-finger nucleases. Proc Natl Acad Sci U S A. 2008;105(15):5809-5814.

[54] Yao X, Wang X, Hu X, Liu Z, Liu J, Zhou H, et al. Homology-mediated end joining-based targeted integration using CRISPR/Cas9. Cell Res. 2017;27(6): 801-814.

[55] Jinek M, Chylinski K, Fonfara I, Hauer M, Doudna JA, Charpentier E. A programmable dual-RNA-guided DNA endonuclease in adaptive bacterial immunity. Science. 2012;337(6096): 816-821.

[56] Ran FA, Hsu PD, Lin CY, Gootenberg JS, Konermann S, Trevino AE, et al. Double nicking by RNA-guided CRISPR Cas9 for enhanced genome editing specificity. Cell. 2013;154(6):1380-1389.

[57] Anzalone AV, Randolph PB, Davis JR, Sousa AA, Koblan LW, Levy JM, et al. Search-and-replace genome editing without double-strand breaks or donor DNA. Nature. 2019;576(7785):149-157.

[58] Bornert O, Hogervorst M, Nauroy P, Bischof J, Swildens J, Athanasiou I, et al. QR-313, an Antisense Oligonucleotide, Shows Therapeutic Efficacy for Treatment of Dominant and Recessive Dystrophic Epidermolysis Bullosa: A Preclinical Study. J Invest Dermatol. 2020. 141(4):883-893.

[59] Koller U, Wally V, Bauer JW, Murauer EM. Considerations for a Successful RNA Trans-splicing Repair of Genetic Disorders. Mol Ther Nucleic Acids. 2014;3:e157.

[60] Chao H, Mansfield SG, Bartel RC, Hiriyanna S, Mitchell LG, Garcia-Blanco MA, et al. Phenotype correction of hemophilia A mice by spliceosome-mediated RNA trans-splicing. Nat Med. 2003;9(8):1015-1019.

[61] Philippi S, Lorain S, Beley C, Peccate C, Precigout G, Spuler S, et al. Dysferlin rescue by spliceosome-mediated pre-mRNA trans-splicing targeting introns harbouring weakly defined 3′ splice sites. Hum Mol Genet. 2015;24(14):4049-4060.

[62] Monjaret F, Bourg N, Suel L, Roudaut C, Le Roy F, Richard I, et al. Cis-splicing and translation of the pre-trans-splicing molecule combine with efficiency in spliceosome-mediated RNA trans-splicing. Mol Ther. 2014; 22(6):1176-1187.

[63] Avale ME, Rodriguez-Martin T, Gallo JM. Trans-splicing correction of tau isoform imbalance in a mouse model of tau mis-splicing. Hum Mol Genet. 2013;22(13):2603-2611.

[64] Atanasova VS, Jiang Q, Prisco M, Gruber C, Pinon Hofbauer J, Chen M, et al. Amlexanox Enhances Premature Termination Codon Read-Through in COL7A1 and Expression of Full Length Type VII Collagen: Potential Therapy for Recessive Dystrophic Epidermolysis Bullosa. J Invest Dermatol. 2017;137(9):1842-1849.

[65] Cogan J, Weinstein J, Wang X, Hou Y, Martin S, South AP, et al. Aminoglycosides restore full-length type VII collagen by overcoming premature termination codons: therapeutic implications for dystrophic epidermolysis bullosa. Mol Ther. 2014;22(10):1741-1752.

[66] Lincoln V, Cogan J, Hou Y, Hirsch M, Hao M, Alexeev V, et al. Gentamicin induces LAMB3 nonsense mutation readthrough and restores functional laminin 332 in junctional epidermolysis bullosa. Proc Natl Acad Sci U S A. 2018;115(28):E6536-E6E45.

[67] Wing K, Sakaguchi S. Regulatory T cells exert checks and balances on self tolerance and autoimmunity. Nat Immunol. 2010;11(1):7-13.

[68] von Boehmer H, Melchers F. Checkpoints in lymphocyte development and autoimmune disease. Nat Immunol. 2010;11(1):14-20.

[69] Prodinger C, Bauer JW, Laimer M. Translational perspectives to treat Epidermolysis bullosa - where do we stand? Exp Dermatol. 2020.

[70] Wally V, Hovnanian A, Ly J, Buckova H, Brunner V, Lettner T, et al. Diacerein orphan drug development for epidermolysis bullosa simplex: A phase 2/3 randomized, placebo-controlled, double-blind clinical trial. J Am Acad Dermatol. 2018;78(5):892-901 e7.

[71] Wally V, Kitzmueller S, Lagler F, Moder A, Hitzl W, Wolkersdorfer M, et al. Topical diacerein for epidermolysis bullosa: a randomized controlled pilot study. Orphanet J Rare Dis. 2013;8:69.

[72] Wally V, Lettner T, Peking P, Peckl-Schmid D, Murauer EM, Hainzl S, et al. The pathogenetic role of IL-1beta in severe epidermolysis bullosa simplex. J Invest Dermatol. 2013;133(7):1901-1903.

[73] Kwong A, Cogan J, Hou Y, Antaya R, Hao M, Kim G, et al. Gentamicin Induces Laminin 332 and Improves Wound Healing in Junctional Epidermolysis Bullosa Patients with Nonsense Mutations. Mol Ther. 2020; 28(5):1327-1338.

[74] Hammersen J, Neuner A, Wild F, Schneider H. Attenuation of Severe Generalized Junctional Epidermolysis Bullosa by Systemic Treatment with Gentamicin. Dermatology. 2019;235(4): 315-322.

[75] Potenzieri C, Undem BJ. Basic mechanisms of itch. Clin Exp Allergy. 2012;42(1):8-19.

[76] Chiou AS, Choi S, Barriga M, Dutt-Singkh Y, Solis DC, Nazaroff J, et al. Phase 2 trial of a neurokinin-1 receptor antagonist for the treatment of chronic itch in patients with epidermolysis bullosa: A randomized clinical trial. J Am Acad Dermatol. 2020;82(6):1415-1421.

[77] Stander S, Spellman MC, Kwon P, Yosipovitch G. The NK1 receptor antagonist serlopitant for treatment of

chronic pruritus. Expert Opin Investig Drugs. 2019;28(8):659-666.

[78] Shehadeh W, Sarig O, Bar J, Sprecher E, Samuelov L. Treatment of epidermolysis bullosa pruriginosa-associated pruritus with dupilumab. Br J Dermatol. 2020;182(6):1495-1497.

[79] Zhou AG, Little AJ, Antaya RJ. Epidermolysis bullosa pruriginosa treated with dupilumab. Pediatr Dermatol. 2020.

[80] Guttmann-Gruber C, Tockner B, Scharler C, Huttner C, Common JE, Tay ASL, et al. Low-dose calcipotriol can elicit wound closure, anti-microbial, and anti-neoplastic effects in epidermolysis bullosa keratinocytes. Sci Rep. 2018; 8(1):13430.

[81] Guttmann-Gruber C, Piñón Hofbauer J, Tockner B, Reichl V, Hofbauer P, Wolkersdorfer M, et al. The impact of low-dose calcipotriol ointment on wound healing, pruritus, and pain in patients with dystrophic epidermolysis bullosa. Acta Derm Venerol. 2020;100:41.

[82] Nystrom A, Bruckner-Tuderman L. Injury- and inflammation-driven skin fibrosis: The paradigm of epidermolysis bullosa. Matrix Biol. 2018;68-69:547-60.

[83] Nystrom A, Thriene K, Mittapalli V, Kern JS, Kiritsi D, Dengjel J, et al. Losartan ameliorates dystrophic epidermolysis bullosa and uncovers new disease mechanisms. EMBO Mol Med. 2015;7(9):1211-1228.

[84] Mittapalli VR, Madl J, Loffek S, Kiritsi D, Kern JS, Romer W, et al. Injury-Driven Stiffening of the Dermis Expedites Skin Carcinoma Progression. Cancer Res. 2016;76(4):940-951.

[85] Fritsch A, Loeckermann S, Kern JS, Braun A, Bosl MR, Bley TA, et al. A hypomorphic mouse model of dystrophic epidermolysis bullosa reveals mechanisms of disease and response to fibroblast therapy. J Clin Invest. 2008;118(5):1669-1679.

[86] Aguado T, Garcia M, Garcia A, Ferrer-Mayorga G, Martinez-Santamaria L, Del Rio M, et al. Raloxifene and n-Acetylcysteine Ameliorate TGF-Signalling in Fibroblasts from Patients with Recessive Dominant Epidermolysis Bullosa. Cells. 2020;9(9).

[87] Mallipeddi R, Wessagowit V, South AP, Robson AM, Orchard GE, Eady RA, et al. Reduced expression of insulin-like growth factor-binding protein-3 (IGFBP-3) in Squamous cell carcinoma complicating recessive dystrophic epidermolysis bullosa. J Invest Dermatol. 2004;122(5):1302-1309.

[88] Kim M, Murrell DF. Update on the pathogenesis of squamous cell carcinoma development in recessive dystrophic epidermolysis bullosa. Eur J Dermatol. 2015;25 Suppl 1:30-32.

[89] Montaudie H, Chiaverini C, Sbidian E, Charlesworth A, Lacour JP. Inherited epidermolysis bullosa and squamous cell carcinoma: a systematic review of 117 cases. Orphanet J Rare Dis. 2016;11(1):117.

[90] Mallipeddi R. Epidermolysis bullosa and cancer. Clin Exp Dermatol. 2002; 27(8):616-623.

[91] Mellerio JE, Robertson SJ, Bernardis C, Diem A, Fine JD, George R, et al. Management of cutaneous squamous cell carcinoma in patients with epidermolysis bullosa: best clinical practice guidelines. Br J Dermatol. 2016; 174(1):56-67.

[92] Cho RJ, Alexandrov LB, den Breems NY, Atanasova VS, Farshchian M, Purdom E, et al. APOBEC mutation drives early-onset squamous cell carcinomas in recessive dystrophic epidermolysis bullosa. Sci Transl Med. 2018;10(455).

[93] Stratigos A, Garbe C, Lebbe C, Malvehy J, del Marmol V, Pehamberger H,

et al. Diagnosis and treatment of invasive squamous cell carcinoma of the skin: European consensus-based interdisciplinary guideline. Eur J Cancer. 2015;51(14):1989-2007.

[94] Maubec E, Petrow P, Scheer-Senyarich I, Duvillard P, Lacroix L, Gelly J, et al. Phase II study of cetuximab as first-line single-drug therapy in patients with unresectable squamous cell carcinoma of the skin. J Clin Oncol. 2011;29(25):3419-3426.

[95] Dai W, Li Y, Zhou Q, Xu Z, Sun C, Tan X, et al. Cetuximab inhibits oral squamous cell carcinoma invasion and metastasis via degradation of epidermal growth factor receptor. J Oral Pathol Med. 2014;43(4):250-257.

[96] Uribe P, Gonzalez S. Epidermal growth factor receptor (EGFR) and squamous cell carcinoma of the skin: molecular bases for EGFR-targeted therapy. Pathol Res Pract. 2011;207(6): 337-342.

[97] Lievre A, Bachet JB, Boige V, Cayre A, Le Corre D, Buc E, et al. KRAS mutations as an independent prognostic factor in patients with advanced colorectal cancer treated with cetuximab. J Clin Oncol. 2008;26(3):374-379.

[98] Diociaiuti A, Steinke H, Nystrom A, Schwieger-Briel A, Meiss F, Pfannenberg C, et al. EGFR inhibition for metastasized cutaneous squamous cell carcinoma in dystrophic epidermolysis bullosa. Orphanet J Rare Dis. 2019;14(1):278.

[99] Arnold AW, Bruckner-Tuderman L, Zuger C, Itin PH. Cetuximab therapy of metastasizing cutaneous squamous cell carcinoma in a patient with severe recessive dystrophic epidermolysis bullosa. Dermatology. 2009;219(1):80-83.

[100] Medek K, Koelblinger P, Koller J, Diem A, Ude-Schoder K, Bauer JW, et al. Wound healing deficits in severe generalized recessive dystrophic epidermolysis bullosa along anticancer treatment with cetuximab. J Dtsch Dermatol Ges. 2019;17(4):448-450.

[101] Owen KL, Brockwell NK, Parker BS. JAK-STAT Signaling: A Double-Edged Sword of Immune Regulation and Cancer Progression. Cancers (Basel). 2019;11(12).

[102] Sen M, Pollock NI, Black J, DeGrave KA, Wheeler S, Freilino ML, et al. JAK kinase inhibition abrogates STAT3 activation and head and neck squamous cell carcinoma tumor growth. Neoplasia. 2015;17(3):256-264.

[103] Jackow J, Rami A, Hayashi R, Hansen C, Guo Z, DeLorenzo D, et al. Targeting the Jak/Signal Transducer and Activator Of Transcription 3 Pathway with Ruxolitinib in a Mouse Model of Recessive Dystrophic Epidermolysis Bullosa-Squamous Cell Carcinoma. J Invest Dermatol. 2020.

[104] Mittapalli VR, Kuhl T, Kuzet SE, Gretzmeier C, Kiritsi D, Gaggioli C, et al. STAT3 targeting in dystrophic epidermolysis bullosa. Br J Dermatol. 2020;182(5):1279-1281.

[105] Watt SA, Pourreyron C, Purdie K, Hogan C, Cole CL, Foster N, et al. Integrative mRNA profiling comparing cultured primary cells with clinical samples reveals PLK1 and C20orf20 as therapeutic targets in cutaneous squamous cell carcinoma. Oncogene. 2011;30(46):4666-4677.

[106] Takai N, Hamanaka R, Yoshimatsu J, Miyakawa I. Polo-like kinases (Plks) and cancer. Oncogene. 2005;24(2):287-291.

[107] Degenhardt Y, Lampkin T. Targeting Polo-like kinase in cancer therapy. Clin Cancer Res. 2010;16(2):384-389.

[108] He X, Xu C. Immune checkpoint signaling and cancer immunotherapy. Cell Res. 2020;30(8):660-669.

[109] Dyck L, Mills KHG. Immune checkpoints and their inhibition in cancer and infectious diseases. Eur J Immunol. 2017;47(5):765-779.

[110] Robert C, Schachter J, Long GV, Arance A, Grob JJ, Mortier L, et al. Pembrolizumab versus Ipilimumab in Advanced Melanoma. N Engl J Med. 2015;372(26):2521-2532.

[111] Chow LQM, Haddad R, Gupta S, Mahipal A, Mehra R, Tahara M, et al. Antitumor Activity of Pembrolizumab in Biomarker-Unselected Patients With Recurrent and/or Metastatic Head and Neck Squamous Cell Carcinoma: Results From the Phase Ib KEYNOTE-012 Expansion Cohort. J Clin Oncol. 2016;34(32):3838-3845.

[112] Migden MR, Rischin D, Schmults CD, Guminski A, Hauschild A, Lewis KD, et al. PD-1 Blockade with Cemiplimab in Advanced Cutaneous Squamous-Cell Carcinoma. N Engl J Med. 2018;379(4):341-351.

[113] Khaddour K, Gorell ES, Dehdashti F, Tang JY, Ansstas G. Induced Remission of Metastatic Squamous Cell Carcinoma with an Immune Checkpoint Inhibitor in a Patient with Recessive Dystrophic Epidermolysis Bullosa. Case Rep Oncol. 2020;13(2):911-915.

Chapter 7

Surgical Treatment of Wounds Using Stem Cells in Epidermolysis Bullosa (EB)

Magdalena Nita, Jacek Pliszczyński, Andrzej Eljaszewicz, Marcin Moniuszko, Tomasz Ołdak, Katarzyna Woźniak, Sławomir Majewski, Cezary Kowalewski, Artur Kamiński, Dariusz Śladowski, Zbigniew Zimek, Maciej Kosieradzki and Piotr Fiedor

Abstract

Epidermolysis bullosa (EB) is a group of hereditary skin diseases, or genodermatoses, characterized by the formation of severe, chronic blisters with painful and life-threatening complications. Despite the previous and ongoing progress in the field, there are still no effective causative treatments for EB. The treatment is limited to relieving symptoms, which—depending on disease severity —may involve skin (blisters, poorly healing wounds caused by the slightest mechanical stimuli, contractures, scarring, pseudosyndactyly) and internal organ abnormalities (esophageal, pyloric, or duodenal atresia; renal failure; and hematopoietic abnormalities). The last decade saw a series of important discoveries that paved the way for new treatment methods, including gene therapy, bone marrow transplantation, cell therapy (allogenic fibroblasts, mesenchymal stem cells [MSCs], and clinical use of induced pluripotent stem cells. Tissue engineering experts are attempting to develop skin-like structures that can facilitate the process of healing to promote skin reconstruction in injuries that are currently incurable. However, this is incredibly challenging, due to the complex structure and the many functions of the skin. Below, we characterize EB and present its potential treatment methods. Despite the cure for EB being still out of reach, recent data from animal models and initial clinical trials in humans have raised patients', clinicians', and researchers' expectations. Consequently, modifying the course of the disease and improving the quality of life have become possible. Moreover, the conclusions drawn based on EB treatment may considerably improve the treatment of other genetic diseases.

Keywords: biological dressing, human skin allograft, allogenic human skin equivalent, Advanced Therapy Medicinal Product, Epidermolysis Bullosa, Rare Diseases

1. Introduction

Epidermolysis Bullosa (EB) is a group of heterogeneous genetic conditions (genodermatoses) characterized by skin fragility and blister formation. These blisters, or bullae, may form spontaneously or as a result of slight mechanical injuries. EB is estimated to occur in 1 person per 50,000 live births.

EB constitutes a group of conditions with diverse clinical courses. Depending on the type of abnormalities in the specific genes, the course, severity, and location of lesions may vary. EB is a result of abnormal connection between the epidermis and dermis. The epidermis, which is the most superficial layer of the skin, constitutes an important barrier between the body and its external environment. The epidermis prevents the loss of water and protects the body against ultraviolet radiation and pathogens. The dermis contains blood vessels, nerve endings, and skin appendages. Under normal conditions, the epidermis and dermis are tightly connected via protein molecules [1–6].

2. The epidermis – structure and functions

The epidermis is the outermost part of the skin and serves as a barrier protecting the body against pathogens, ultraviolet radiation, and excessive loss of water. The epidermal layers, listed from the deepest to the most superficial, include the basal, spinous, granular, and cornified layers. The basal layer is composed of keratinocytes, which undergo intense cell divisions. The newly formed cells differentiate as they progress towards the epidermal surface, eventually becoming dead, anuclear cells (corneocytes) that have no mitochondria. Since they are surrounded by a lipid layer, corneocytes form an impermeable barrier. The epidermis is strongly and permanently connected to the dermis via a cytoskeleton and hemidesmosomes. (**Figure 1**) [7–9].

The course of EB may be severe if the condition is due to a lack of key adhesion proteins, for example as a result of loss-of-function mutations in laminin 332 or collagen VII genes. Conversely, isolated amino acid substitutions typically lead to a mild fragility of the skin. The genetic and allelic heterogeneity of EB is due to

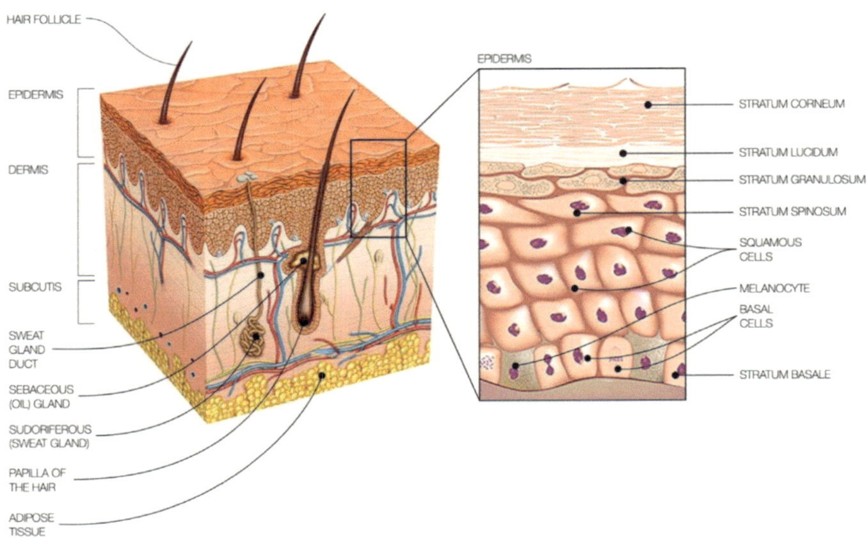

Figure 1.
Skin structure. (from private sources MN).

pathological gene variants in 20 different genes. The genes associated with EB encode intracellular, transmembrane, or extracellular proteins that constitute structural components of the cytoskeleton (keratin 5 and 14), extracellular matrix (integrin α6β4, collagen XVII, laminin 332, collagen VII, α3 integrin, kindlin-1), or intercellular adhesions (desmoplakin, plakophilin, plakoglobin).

3. Epidermolysis Bullosa

The key clinical manifestation of EB is a tendency to develop skin lesions in response to mechanical stimuli, even those of a very low magnitude. The most common lesion types include blisters, milia, pigmented lesions, erosions, epidermal defects, and scars. Other characteristic features of the condition are nail plate changes, ranging from dystrophy to a complete loss. Another common symptom is hair loss and—in severe cases—alopecia. Blisters, erosions, and scars developing near joints may result in contractures and tissue adhesions due to scarring. The lesions that develop on hands and feet (which are most prone to mechanical injuries) may result in pseudosyndactyly. Contractures exacerbate hand and foot deformities, leading to disability ("cocoon hand", or "mitten hand" deformities).

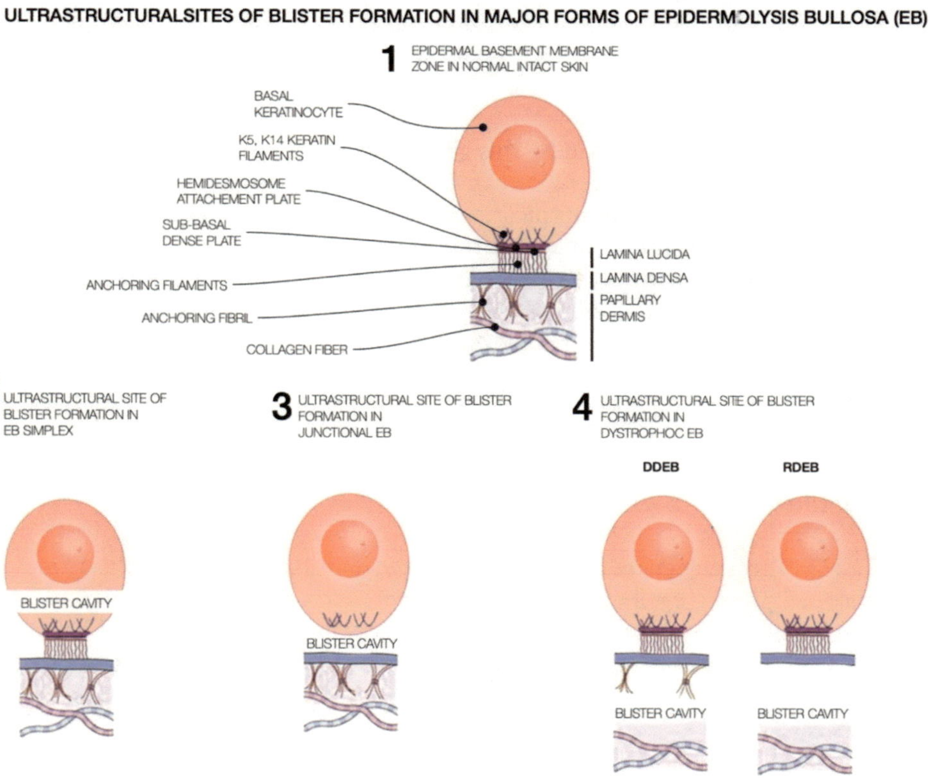

Figure 2.
Ultrastructural sites of blister formation in major forms of epidermolysis bullosa EB. 1. In intact skin, the ultrastructural regions of the epidermal basement membrane zone consist of basal keratinocytes and the hemodesmosomal plaque, the lamina lucida, the lamina densa, the upper papillary dermis 2. in eb simplex (EBS), blisters arise within the lower portion of basal keratinocytes 3. In junctional EB (JEB) blisters form within the lamina lucida 4. In dystrophic EB (DEB), blisters develop below the lamina densa. Anchoring fibris are reduced in number in dominant DEB (DDEB) and absent or rudimentary in recessive DEB (RDEB). KRT5,KRT14 and keratin 5 and keratin14 respectively (s. https://plasticsurgerykey.com/epidermolysis-bullosa/).

Severe forms of EB additionally involve internal anomalies in the oral cavity, esophagus, trachea, lungs, urinary catheter, or urinary bladder. Intestinal tract erosions, ulcerations, and scarring lead to strictures, which may result in difficulty swallowing (dysphagia) and necessitate a feeding jenunostomy to provide enteral nutrition. Oral manifestations of EB may include the tongue adhering to the floor of the mouth (ankyloglossia); a narrowed oral opening (microstomia); and difficulties in chewing and swallowing, which result in malnourishment, osteopenia, osteoporosis, growth retardation, and eating disorders, leading to cachexia. Oral lesions may cause oral hygiene problems, which leads to caries. Perianal erosions and ulcerations cause severe pain during defecation, which contributes to constipation. Possible ocular manifestations involve marginal blepharitis, eyelash loss, ectropion, adhesions between the palpebral and bulbar conjunctivae (symblepharon), and corneal blistering, which may lead to blindness. Other manifestations include treatment-refractory anemia, iron deficiency, and hypoalbuminemia. Due to chronic ulcerations and an impaired protective function of the epidermis, EB patients may develop skin cancer (squamous cell carcinoma [SCC]) in their thirties or forties (**Figure 2**) [10–15].

3.1 Classification

EB is a result of mutations in approximately 20 genes that encode structural and enzymatic proteins responsible for forming and maintaining the connections between the epidermis and dermis. The most common mutations occur in one of three genes: *KRT5*, *KRT14*, or *TGM5*.

- KRT5: The protein encoded by this gene is a member of the keratin gene family. The type II cytokeratins consist of basic or neutral proteins which are arranged in pairs of heterotypic keratin chains coexpressed during differentiation of simple and stratified epithelial tissues. This type II cytokeratin is specifically expressed in the basal layer of the epidermis with family member KRT14. Mutations in these genes have been associated with a complex of diseases termed epidermolysis bullosa simplex. The type II cytokeratins are clustered in a region of chromosome 12q12-q13. (RefSeq, Jul 2008)

- KRT14: This gene product, a type I keratin. At least one pseudogene has been identified at 17p12-p11.

- TGM5: This gene encodes a member of the transglutaminase family. The encoded protein catalyzes formation of protein cross-links between glutamine and lysine residues, often resulting in stabilization of protein assemblies. This reaction is calcium dependent. Mutations in this gene have been associated with acral peeling skin syndrome (RefSeq, Oct 2009). [https://www.genecards.org/]

EB can be classified into three main types, which can be further divided into subtypes. This classification is based on anomalies in various protein molecules and each of the resulting EB types has a different clinical course.

- simple epidermolysis bullosa (SEB) involves epidermal anomalies

- junctional epidermolysis bullosa (JEB) involves basement membrane anomalies

DOI: http://dx.doi.org/10.5772/intechopen.97036

- dystrophic epidermolysis bullosa (DEB) involves anomalies of the dermis

The diagnosis is made based on a thorough microscopic examination of a skin sample. The examination helps determine the exact layer of the skin where tissue separation causes blister formation. There are several layers that can be identified under a microscope in a skin cross-section. If the blisters form within the epidermis, the patient is diagnosed with SEB; if they form within the lamina lucida, the patient is diagnosed with JEB, and if they form just underneath the lamina densa, the patient is diagnosed with DEB (**Table 1**).

Overview of EB classification			
Subtype	**Phenotype**	**Inheritance**	**Gene affected**
EB simplex — Intraepidermal			
EB simplex, localized	Palmoplantar blistering from birth or early infancy, with subsequent keratoderma in affected areas	AD	*KRT5 or KRT14*
EB simplex, severe	Early generalized blistering at or soon after birth; congenital areas of denuded skin may be present; can be life threatening in first year of life; classically, tense clustered 'herpetiform' blisters arise with minimal trauma or spontaneously; development of confluent palmoplantar keratoderma; nail dystrophy common	AD	*KRT5 or KRT14*
EB simplex, intermediate	Generalized, although less severe blistering than EB simplex, severe	AD	*KRT5 or KRT14*
EB simplex with mottled pigmentation	Blistering from birth of intermediate severity; additional mottled or reticulate macular pigmentation typically of the neck, upper trunk and acral skin; punctate keratoderma; nail dystrophy may develop	AD	*Predominantly KRT5; less frequently KRT14*
EB simplex, migratory circinate	Vesicles from birth, on a background of inflammatory migratory circinate erythema that fades to leave post-inflammatory hyperpigmentation; nail dystrophy possible	AD	*KRT5*
EB simplex, intermediate with cardiomyopathy	Marked erosions in limbs at birth, healing with dyspigmentation and atrophic burn-like scars; keratoderma, nail-thickening and onychogryphosis possible; diffuse alopecia has occasionally been reported; dilated cardiomyopathy develops later in young adulthood	AD	*KLHL24*
EB simplex, intermediate with PLEC mutations	*Autosomal dominant disease is mild with mainly acral blistering; autosomal recessive has an intermediate presentation*	AD or AR	*PLEC*
EB simplex, intermediate with muscular dystrophy	Generalized blistering with variable-onset myopathy including possible cardiomyopathy; focal plantar	AR	*PLEC*

Overview of EB classification			
Subtype	**Phenotype**	**Inheritance**	**Gene affected**
	keratoderma and nail dystrophy; mucosal involvement is common; upper respiratory tract stenosis has been reported		
EB simplex, severe with pyloric atresia	More severe, widespread generalized blistering or loss of skin at birth with pyloric atresia; early mortality within a few months of birth	AR	*PLEC*
EB simplex, autosomal recessive, KRT5 or KRT14	Generalized blistering, intermediate or severe; keratin 5 abnormalities tend to have a more severe phenotype; absence of keratin 5 associated with widespread skin disease and early mortality; improvement of blistering with age is not expected	AR	*KRT5 or KRT14*
EB simplex, localized or intermediate with BP230 deficiency	Early-onset blistering, relatively mild, usually with acral predominance; plantar keratoderma	AR	*DST*
EB simplex, localized or intermediate with exophilin 5 deficiency	Generalized intermittent blistering and skin fragility; mild mottled pigmentation may be evident	AR	*EXPH5*
EB simplex, localized with nephropathy (CD151 deficiency)	Early blistering, with pretibial predominance; poikiloderma may be seen; early alopecia; extracutaneous involvement manifests as oesophageal webbing and nephropathy	AR	*CD151*
Junctional EB, severe	Blistering may be mild at birth and localized to periungual, buttock and elbow regions; overgranulation develops, particularly on orofacial and periungual regions, with development of bulbous nail folds; alopecia is common; dental enamel defects are usual; a hoarse cry is often a feature; usually fatal within the first 2 years of life	AR	*LAMA3, LAMB3 and LAMC2*
Junctional EB, intermediate	Less severe than above, with a reduced tendency to develop exuberant granulation tissue; elevated risk of SCC in adulthood	AR	*LAMA3, LAMB3, LAMC2 and COL17A*
Junctional EB with pyloric atresia	Extensive areas of skin loss seen at birth with severe cutaneous fragility; early-onset pyloric atresia, a frequent cause of early mortality, within days or weeks of birth; duodenal and anal atresia may also feature; milder non-lethal variants often show genitourinary involvement	AR	*ITGA6 and ITG84*
Junctional EB, localized	Limited cutaneous fragility, often acral; variable nail and dental defects; normal hair	AR	*LAMA3, LAMB3, LAMC2, COL17A1, ITGB4 and ITGA3*

Overview of EB classification			
Subtype	**Phenotype**	**Inheritance**	**Gene affected**
Junctional EB, inversa	Flexural blistering from birth; dental abnormalities and nail loss	AR	*LAMA3, LAMB3 and LAMC2*
Junctional EB, late onset	Onset in childhood, with often acral fragility; skin fragility is progressive and loss of dermatoglyphs may be seen owing to scarring; variable dental enamel and nail defects	AR	*COL17A1*
Junctional EB–laryngo-onycho-cutaneous (LOC) syndrome	Skin fragility from birth with marked exuberant granulation tissue (greater than that in junctional EB, severe), particularly on face and neck; nail dystrophy and loss with granulation tissue of nail beds; laryngeal granulation can lead to respiratory compromise and death; conjunctival and eyelid granulation with consequent symblepharon, scarring and visual loss	AR	*LAMA3*
Junctional EB with interstitial lung disease and nephrotic syndrome	Variable degree of cutaneous involvement; fatality in early childhood is common; nail dystrophy possible; hair loss may occur	AR	*IGTA3*
Dystrophic EB — sublamina densa			
Intermediate $DDEB_1$	Generalized skin fragility, scarring and milia presenting from birth or early infancy, with prominence over acral sites, elbows and knees; involvement of the mucous membranes may lead to microstomia, ankyloglossia and oesophageal stenosis, although less commonly than in severe RDEB	AD	*COL7A1*
Localized $DDEB_1$	Predominantly acral blistering, scarring and milia seen from birth or early infancy; occasional nails-only presentation, with progressive dystrophy and eventual nail loss; rarely, cutaneous features may predominate over pretibial skin alone (and can present as late-onset disease)	AD	*COL7A1*
DDEB, $pruriginosa_1$	Profoundly pruritic linear cords of papules associated with fragility, scarring and milia on the shins, and occasionally progressing to arms; may present in childhood or adulthood; nail dystrophy is usual	AD	*COL7A1*
DDEB, self-$improving_{1,2}$	Blistering evident at or shortly after birth, usually on extremities where there may be aplasia cutis, whilst scarring and milia may occur; spontaneous resolution of cutaneous fragility within the first 2 years of life	AD	*COL7A1*

Overview of EB classification			
Subtype	**Phenotype**	**Inheritance**	**Gene affected**
Intermediate RDEB3	Phenotype similar to that of intermediate DDEB, although greater severity with flexion contractures, limited digital fusion and occasional striate keratoderma	AR	*COL7A1*
Severe RDEB3	Widespread blistering from birth, with extensive scarring and development of microstomia, ankyloglossia, oesophageal stenosis, flexion contractures of limbs and pseudosyndactyly; nails are often lost early in disease course; high risk of cutaneous SCC arising in EB wounds.	AR	*COL7A1*
RDEB, inversa3	Generalized blistering from birth, of intermediate severity; subsequently, fragility tends to be displayed on flexural sites	AR	*COL7A1*
RDEB, localized3	Skin fragility and blistering typically at birth or neonatal period, limited to acral sites such as hands and feet, or occasionally only to pretibial skin, where it may manifest as late-onset disease during adulthood; nail dystrophy and loss usual	AR	*COL7A1*
RDEB, pruriginosa3	As for DDEB, pruriginosa	AR	*COL7A1*
RDEB, self-improving3	As for DDEB, self-improving	AR	*COL7A1*
DEB, severe4	Clinically indistinguishable from severe RDEB, with severe mucocutaneous fragility from birth	Dominant and recessive compound heterozygosity	*COL7A1*
Kindler EB — variable and mixed			
None	Generalized blistering and variable photosensitivity from birth or early childhood, with mucosal fragility; blistering gives way to progressive poikiloderma, initially most marked over dorsal hands and neck; confluent palmoplantar keratoderma and adermatoglyphia may occur; gingivitis and dental disease is a feature; oesophageal narrowing and colitis has been reported; mucocutaneous SCC has been reported, with poor prognosis	*AR*	*FERMT1*

AD, autosomal dominant; AR, autosomal recessive; DDEB, dominant dystrophic epidermolysis bullosa; DEB; dystrophic epidermolysis bullosa; EB, epidermolysis bullosa; EM, electron microscopy; ER, endoplasmic reticulum; RDEB, recessive dystrophic epidermolysis bullosa; SCC, squamous cell carcinoma. 1Major type is DDEB. 2Previously known as transient bullous dermolysis of the newborn baby. 3Major type is RDEB. 4Major type is DEB (dominant and recessive compound heterotygosity). Adapted from consensus guidelines3.

Table 1.
Overview of EB classification [16].

3.2 Heredity

SEB primarily shows an autosomal dominant pattern of inheritance, with the most common mutations in genes *KRT5* and *KRT14*. Autosomal recessive inheritance is less common and caused by mutations in genes *KRT14*, *ITGA6*, *ITGB4* (*this genes encodes a member of the integrin alpha chain family of proteins. Integrins are heterodimeric integral membrane proteins composed of an alpha chain and a beta chain that function in cell surface adhesion and signaling. The encoded preproprotein is proteolytically processed to generate light and heavy chains that comprise the alpha 6 subunit. This subunit may associate with a beta 1 or beta 4 subunit to form an integrin that interacts with extracellular matrix proteins including members of the laminin family. The alpha 6 beta 4 integrin may promote tumorigenesis, while the alpha 6 beta 1 integrin may negatively regulate erbB2/HER2 signaling. Alternative splicing results in multiple transcript variants. [provided by RefSeq, Oct 2015]*).

DSP (This gene encodes a protein that anchors intermediate filaments to desmosomal plaques and forms an obligate component of functional desmosomes), or *PKP1 (Plakophilin proteins contain numerous armadillo repeats, localize to cell desmosomes and nuclei, and participate in linking cadherins to intermediate filaments in the cytoskeleton. This protein may be involved in molecular recruitment and stabilization during desmosome formation)*. SEB caused by a *PLEC1(Plakins, with their multi-domain structure and enormous size, not only play crucial roles in maintaining cell and tissue integrity and orchestrating dynamic changes in cytoarchitecture and cell shape, but also serve as scaffolding platforms for the assembly, positioning, and regulation of signaling complexes (reviewed in PMID: 9701547, 11854008, and 17499243)* mutation may show an autosomal recessive or autosomal dominant pattern of inheritance.

JEB is primarily caused by mutations in genes *LAMB3, LAMC2, LAMA3 (this genes is a laminin that belongs to a family of basement membrane proteins), COL17A1* (This gen encode *collagen XVII is a structural component of hemidesmosomes, multiprotein complexes at the dermal-epidermal basement membrane zone that mediate adhesion of keratinocytes to the underlying membrane), ITGA*6 or *ITGB4* and is characterized by autosomal recessive inheritance. A recent study (2009) showed a possible autosomal dominant inheritance pattern in the case of a mutated *COL17A1*.

DEB is caused by mutations in only one gene, *COLA1*. The location and type of mutation determine the inheritance pattern (autosomal recessive or dominant).

3.3 SEB subtypes

- Koebner type: mutated genes for keratin 5 and 4 (*KRT5*, *KRT4*); lesions are often present at birth or in infancy; characteristic features are hyperkeratotic lesions, hemorrhagic bullae, and erosions.

- Dowling-Meara type: mutated *KRT14* and *KRT5* genes, which encode keratin 14 and 5, respectively; autosomal dominant inheritance; lesions are located primarily on the feet, less commonly in other locations; a relatively mild course.

- Weber-Cockayne type: associated with mutated *KRT5* (region 12q13.13) and *KRT14* (region 17q21.2) genes; characterized by a severe course and herpetiform blisters. Poorly healing blisters and erosions lead to scarring and contractures.

- SEB with muscular dystrophy: a mutated plectin-encoding *PLEC1* gene.

3.4 JEB subtypes

- JEB with pyloric atresia: this rare type of EB results from mutated *ITGB4* and *ITGA6* genes that encode α6 β4 integrin. Skin lesions are accompanied by esophageal, pyloric, and/or duodenal atresia. Enamel hypoplasia is common.

- Herlitz type: mutations in the *LAMA3*, *LAMB3*, and *LAMC2* genes, which encode the polypeptide subunits of laminin 5 (α-3, β-3, and γ-2, respectively). Fatal type of EB, characterized by blisters and erosions over the entire body, which causes multiple infections that may lead to sepsis, loss of proteins (malnourishment), scarring, contractures, defects of large areas of skin.

- Non-Herlitz type: mutations in genes *COL17A1*, *LAMB3*, *LAMC2*, or *LAMA3* encoding laminin 5 and collagen XVII.

3.5 DEB subtypes

- Hallopeau-Siemens type: a mutated *COL7A1* gene, which encodes collagen VII. This type of EB is characterized by scarring, erosions, pseudosyndactyly of the hands and feet; nail plate involvement, esophageal atresia, and corneal ulcers are common.

- non-Hallopeau-Siemens type: mutated *COL7A1* gene, encoding collagen VII.

- Cockayne-Toureine type: autosomal dominant inheritance; mutated *COL7A1* (collagen VII); skin lesion on the limbs.

- Pasini type: possible nail plate involvement; oral and mucosal lesions.

3.6 Diagnostic investigations

A primary diagnosis of EB is based on the clinical presentation. The definitive diagnosis is established after skin samples are examined via immunofluorescence antigen mapping and transmission microscopy.

Diagnosis is confirmed via genetic analysis that determines the type of mutation.

3.7 Differential diagnoses

The differential diagnoses should include congenital dermatoses, herpes simplex virus infections, epidermolytic hyperkeratosis with erosions and blisters, staphylococcal scalded skin syndrome, bullous pemphigoid, neonatal pemphigoid, and gestational pemphigoid.

3.8 Treatment

Management is primarily symptomatic. Surgical treatment mainly involves skin grafting. Importantly, the use of autologous skin grafts is ineffective due to poor healing and chronic wound formation at the donor sites. Plastic surgery procedures play an important role in repairing contractures and pseudosyndactyly of the hands and feet. In the case of esophageal, pyloric or duodenal atresia, various surgical procedures are used to overcome the effects of gastrointestinal strictures (e.g. feeding jejunostomy, endoscopic balloon dilatation).

EB management involves primarily local care of chronic wounds, ulcers, erosions, and blisters. Treatment challenges involve frequent bacterial infections, due to their chronic character, and factors that inhibit healing, such as malnutrition, anemia, itching, or repetitive wound irritation with regular dressing changes, all of which disturb epithelialization. Moreover, wounds may cause severe pain, exacerbated by regular, frequent dressing changes. Importantly, the condition requires life-long care, with the cost of monthly treatment often exceeding several hundred dollars. Therefore, the process of selecting the optimal dressing should include the following parameters: the price, availability, effectiveness, and safety. Other important complementary treatments include physiotherapy, genetic counselling, aggressive treatment of infections, nutritional supplementation, and skin cancer monitoring [17–31].

Despite the enormous advances in our understanding of molecular genetics and EB physiopathology that have taken place over the last several decades, a definitive cure is yet to be discovered. There are many ongoing studies aiming to develop an effective treatment. These studies focus on several potential lines of treatment, including disease modifying treatments to diminish disease severity. Gene therapies, bone marrow transplants, and tissue engineering are receiving the most attention.

Advanced therapy medicinal products (ATMPs) are medicines for human use that are based on genes, tissues or cells. They offer groundbreaking new opportunities for the treatment of disease and injury. ATMPs can be classified into three main types: gene therapy medicines, somatic-cell therapy medicines, tissue-engineered medicines. In addition, some ATMPs may contain one or more medical devices as an integral part of the medicine, which are referred to as combined ATMPs. An example of this is cells embedded in a biodegradable matrix or scaffold.

Gene therapy involves cultures of keratinocytes (obtained from patients with recessive DEB [RDEB]) that have been transduced with a retroviral vector containing full-length cDNA of the *COL7A1* gene (for collagen VII). These cultures are, subsequently, placed onto the patient's wounds in the form of epidermal grafts [32]. Treatment efficacy and collagen VII expression were demonstrated; however, the response lasted up to 12 months. Nonetheless this therapy is safe. One disadvantage of this method is the fact that it can be used in limited areas (at chronic wound sites). This method has been also used in a patient with JEB, in whom the placement of genetically corrected keratinocytes onto chronic wound sites led to successful wound healing. Based on the available reports, gene therapies are promising treatment modalities with a potential therapeutic effect in genodermatoses.

Bone marrow transplant (BMT) and allogenic stem cell transplantation (ASCT) are other very promising treatment strategies. In 2010, Wagner et al. performed ASCT in children with RDEB. Although the patients were not completely cured, their skin blisters were reduced, and skin regeneration was accelerated. BMT in RDEB patients has been reported to improve the clinical status, despite the lack of collagen VII growth in the skin. BMT is an experimental therapy, which is used as part of clinical studies, and currently is not an approved treatment. The risk of death and the uncertain degree and mechanism of the clinical response should be viewed in light of the results of the most recent translational research in RDEB, which reports ASCT to be currently the only therapeutic approach that shows systemic effects in what essentially is a systemic disease. There is a clear need for reports presenting data from extensive clinical studies to establish guidelines and warnings for the use of ASCT in EB treatment.

As pluripotent cells, MSCs have a potential to differentiate into many different types of skin cells, including keratinocytes, endothelial cells, and monocytes. Due to their immunomodulatory and anti-inflammatory effects, MSCs may play a significant role in wound healing and tissue regeneration. Moreover, MSCs do not trigger an immune response in the recipient, hence there is no need to match the donor's and recipient's human leukocyte antigen (HLA) types [33]. Due to their multi-directional differentiation potential, MSCs have been shown to regenerate collagen VII, which has a beneficial effect on the healing of wounds (including chronic wounds) and improves skin stability. These effects were observed with intradermal administration, which—apart from presenting fewer challenges—does not require as many MSCs as intravenous administration. Most studies have focused on bone marrow-derived MSCs (BM-MSCs). However, their harvesting from the bone marrow is a relatively invasive procedure. Moreover, the multipotent differentiation potential of BM-MSCs diminishes with age. Therefore, MSCs are currently obtained from alternative sources, such as the umbilical cord [34], which can provide up to a billion cells in 30 days, obtained non-invasively. The umbilical cord consists of umbilical vessels surrounded by a connective tissue, referred to as Wharton jelly (WJ). WJ-derived MSCs have a higher proliferative potential and are more homogeneous than those derived from the bone marrow. WJ-MSCs are similar to BM-MSCs in their fibroblast-like phenotype, non-hematopoietic surface markers [35], low immunogenicity [36], multipotent plasticity, and the expression of CD90, CD73, CD105 markers [37]. Moreover, WJ-MSCs seem to have more pronounced pro-angiogenic properties than BM-MSCs; they promote neovascularization and perfusion by releasing paracrine factors and by playing the role of perivascular precursor cells [38]. WJ-MSCs are a highly efficient source of young, non-carcinogenic, and non-immunomodulatory cells [39]. All these properties and the fact that WJ-MSCs are easily available make these cells a promising strategy for treating wounds in EB patients.

Sebastiano et al. propose an innovating cell therapy for RDEB treatment, by developing a state of the art protocol of genetically repaired induced pluripotent stem cells (iPSCs) as to generate sheets of normal skin tissue to treat affected skin areas [40]. Moreover, as numerous stem cells are needed in order to cover the affected surface area, authors outline the necessity for creating personalized iPSCs banks as to provide a constant long-term iPSCs source. Generally, human iPSCs can be generated by reprogramming differentiated somatic cells into pluripotent embryonic stem cells (ESCs) capable of differentiating into ectoderm, mesoderm or endoderm cells. Reprogramming involves the introduction of a known set of genes into the somatic cells, using integrating viral and non-integrating non-viral methods. Following successful reprogramming, somatic cells will express genes and surface proteins similar to ESCs in vitro and will be able to differentiate into any of the three embryonic germ layers.

Tissue engineering: Not unlike patients with extensive burns, patients with EB do not qualify for autologous skin grafts. One solution available to these patients involves the use of allogeneic grafts, which serve to temporarily cover the wound (after 7 days the graft is rejected by the recipient; [41]). Therefore, tissue engineering seems to be a promising solution, as it helps create biopolymer scaffolds to cover the wounds. The idea is to create skin substitutes, which can then be seeded with keratinocytes, fibroblasts, or stem cells. Such polymer materials constitute a micro-environment and provide adequate scaffolds for cell colonization and epithelial cell migration during wound epithelialization. The multi-disciplinary nature of tissue engineering has helped develop many bioengineered skin substitutes, with potential applications as a suitable dressing for treating refractory wounds, such as those in EB patients. The field of tissue engineering has been rapidly transferring from the realm of basic research to commercial applications. There are many in vitro-generated skin substitutes. They are available in various forms, which include epidermal, dermal, and dermo-epidermal analogs or complex skin analogs, and can be composed of cellular or acellular scaffolds [42–51].

High-quality, safe skin analogs should be cost-effective, biocompatible, biodegradable, and noncarcinogenic, carry no risk of infectious disease transfer, and provoke no activation of the recipient's immune system. Despite a whole spectrum of bioengineered products currently available on the market, there are scarcely any that meet all the requirements of natural skin. Natural skin is composed of the epidermis, dermis, and subcutaneous tissue. It contains appendages, such as sweat glands, nails, and hair, as well as nerve endings and blood vessels. Additionally, natural skin protects the body against the external environment via its thermoregulatory function and its role in maintaining water–electrolyte balance. It also facilitates the perception of pain, heat, and touch; manufactures vitamin D; and shields the body against ultraviolet radiation by the means of melanin-producing melanocytes responsible for skin pigmentation [52, 53]. Due to the wide range of functions performed by human skin, creating its analog is a challenge for tissue engineers.

The first product that has transferred the potential of bioengineering into real-life EB applications is an autologous cultured epidermal substitute (CES). The pioneering study by Rheinwald and Green demonstrated that epidermal keratinocytes from a single-cell suspension can be cultured in the form of sheets, and the resulting multi-layered sheets have proven to be very effective in the treatment of burns and wounds in EB patients. There are many commercially available skin substitutes composed of both epidermal and dermal components. Bell et al. developed a cultured skin substitute (CSS) (an equivalent of living skin) composed of keratinocytes and fibroblasts in a collagen gel. Boyce and Hansbrough developed a CSS composed of a collagen-glycosaminoglycan composite scaffold populated with keratinocytes and fibroblasts. Kuroyanagi et al. developed another CSS, composed of a spongy collagen matrix with keratinocytes and fibroblasts. Such two-layered CSSs are intended to permanently cover full-thickness skin defects. There have been studies on wound healing in EB with the use of OrCelTM, Biobrane, and Apligraf dressings. OrCelTM is a bilayer dressing composed of a bovine-collagen I matrix populated with neonatal foreskin keratinocytes and fibroblasts [54–56]. Despite the fact that OrCelTM exhibits beneficial wound healing properties in RDEB patients—via cytokines and growth factors, such as tumor growth factor alpha (TGFα), fibroblast growth factor 1 (FGF-1), and keratinocyte growth factor 1 (KGF-1)—its bovine collagen component increases the risk of graft rejection and transfer of diseases to the donor [57]. Another bilayer skin substitute is Biobrane, which is composed of a 3D nylon fiber scaffold and an ultrathin semipermeable epidermis-mimicking silicone layer that controls fluid loss [56–59]. The nylon fibers are surrounded by porcine collagen type 1. Jutkiewicz and Noszczyk [60] were the first to report the use of Biobrane in the postoperative hand care in a group of RDEB patients. Apligraf is another bilayer skin substitute composed of dermal and epidermal analogs. The epidermal and dermal layers contain cultured keratinocytes and neonatal foreskin fibroblasts. The dermal layer additionally contains bovine collagen type 1, which facilitates cell growth and differentiation. Apligraf has a short life span, and its use is associated with high costs [57]. Nonetheless, this dressing was reported to be effective in treating EB wounds [61, 62].

Safe and Effective Therapy in the Light of Clinical Trials - New Approach to Treatment by Innovative Method (BIOOPA-ATMP) grant no. STRATERMED2/269807/14/NCBR/2015.

Alternative promising product for the treatment of chronic wounds that occur in EB and other genodermatoses, as well as in burns, is an allogeneic, acellular human skin equivalent sterilized with radiation, and seeded with Wharton's jelly-derived mesenchymal stem cells- WJ-MSCs about the acronym in polish BIOOPA (biological dressing) is an advanced therapy medicinal product composed of a decellularized matrix of the superficial layers of cadaveric human skin (10 cm × 10 cm). Acellular dermal matrix (ADM) is a Chemically/enzymatically processed allograft. This processing removes all epidermal and dermal cells while preserving the molecular and physiological structure of collagen fibers. The scaffold is sterilized via radiation and then seeded with 30 million WJ-MSCs. As a result of decellularization, this skin substitute does not induce an immune response in the recipient and poses a lower risk of transmitting any diseases. In order to assess the safety and efficacy of the BIOOPA dressing, the relevant study was conducted in two stages. During the first stage, in vitro experiments showed BIOOPA viability. All examination techniques demonstrated graft infiltration by host cells and neovascularization of the biological dressing. Moreover, BIOOPA is characterized by low immunogenicity, which was confirmed in histopathology examinations and in vitro T-cell proliferation tests. The second stage of the study was conducted in a group of qualified volunteers with EB and approved by an ethics committee. The 6-month follow-up indicates the safety and efficacy of the BIOOPA dressing, with no infections or necrosis at the graft implantation site observed over the follow-up period. The subjects reported decreased pain and improved quality of life **Figures 3–8** [63, 64].

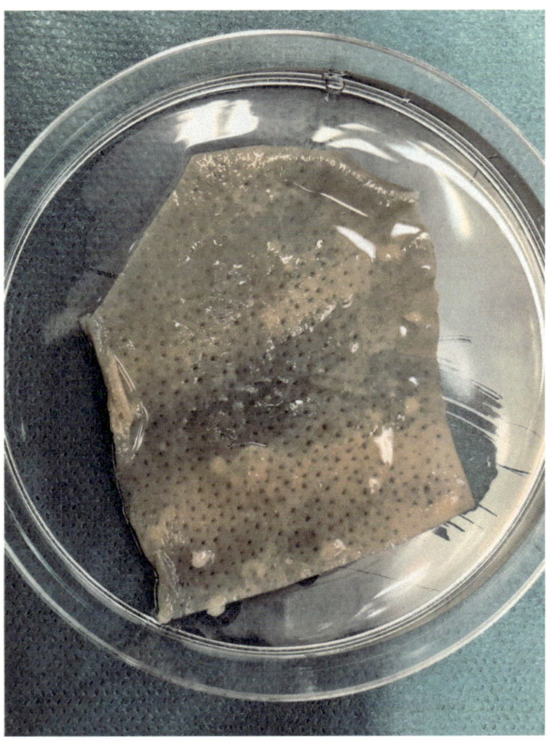

Figure 3.
BIOOPA- Advanced Therapy Medicinal Product (ATMP) acellular human skin equivalent sterilized with ultraviolet radiation.

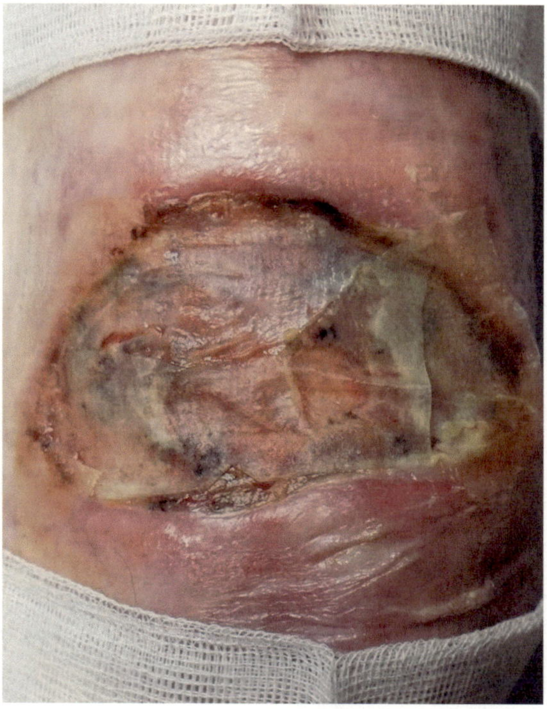

Figure 4.
Day 0, procedure: chronic wound in the knee area covered with prepared graft in the 20-years old patient with EB (allogenic,acellular, human skin equivalent).

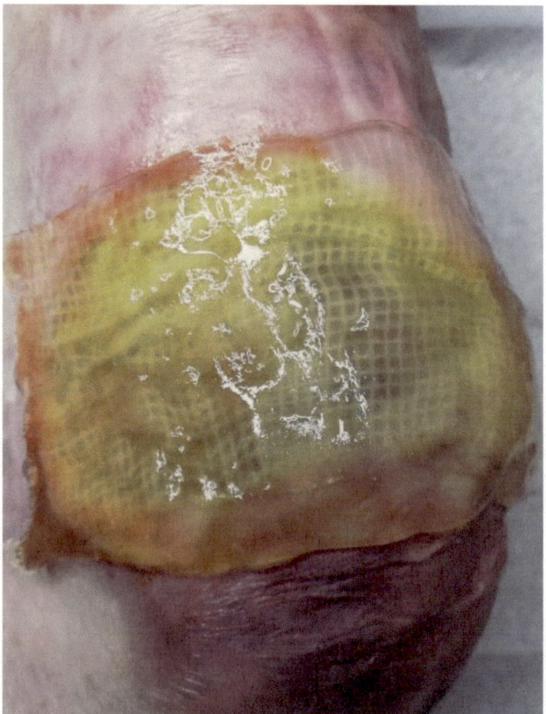

Figure 5.
Bioopa dressing: The scaffold is seeded with 30 million WJ-MSCs in 5 mL of a 5% human albumin solution covered with chlorhexidine-impregnated dressings and collagen gel. The same 20-years old patient with EB (chronic wound in the knee area).

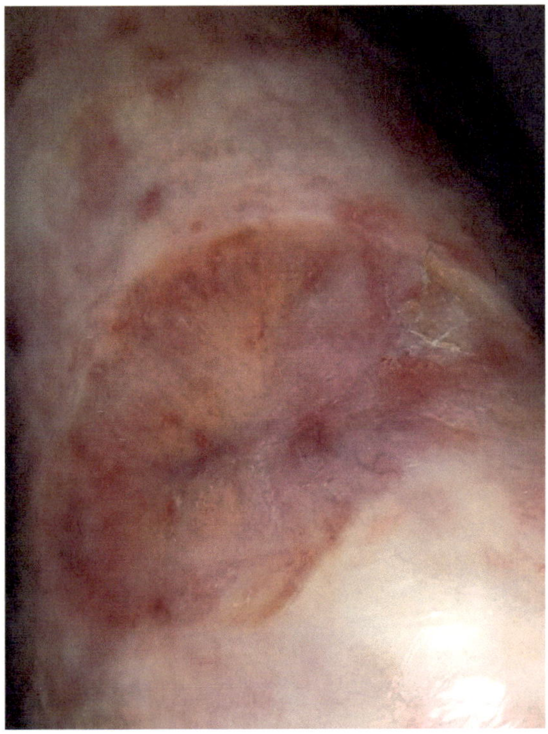

Figure 6.
Results after 30-day follow-up in this patient with EB: All examination techniques revealed host-cell infiltration and neovascularization of the biological dressing. They are characterized by low immunogenicity, as confirmed by histopathology and in vitro T-cell proliferation assays.

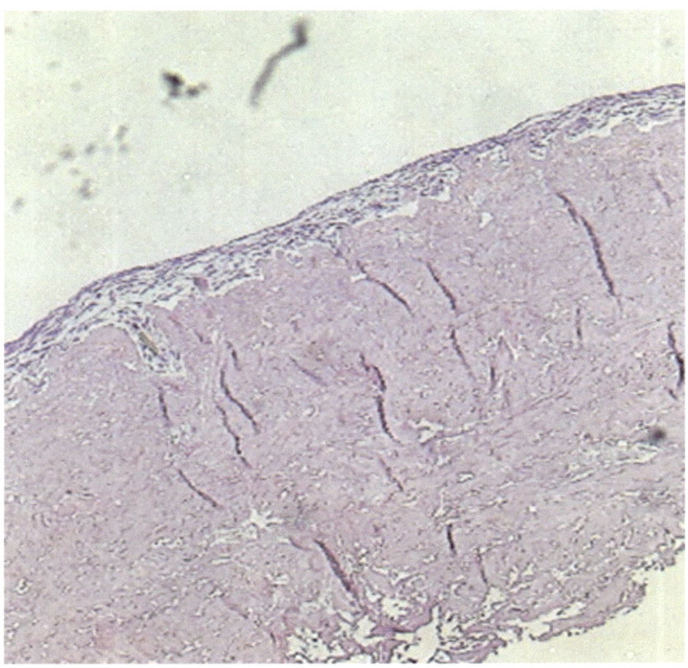

Figure 7.
Hematoxylin and eosin stain of scaffold populated with mesenchymal cells from Wharton's jelly. After 72 hours of culture mesenchymal stem cells create a multilayer structure on the scaffold resembling human epithelium.

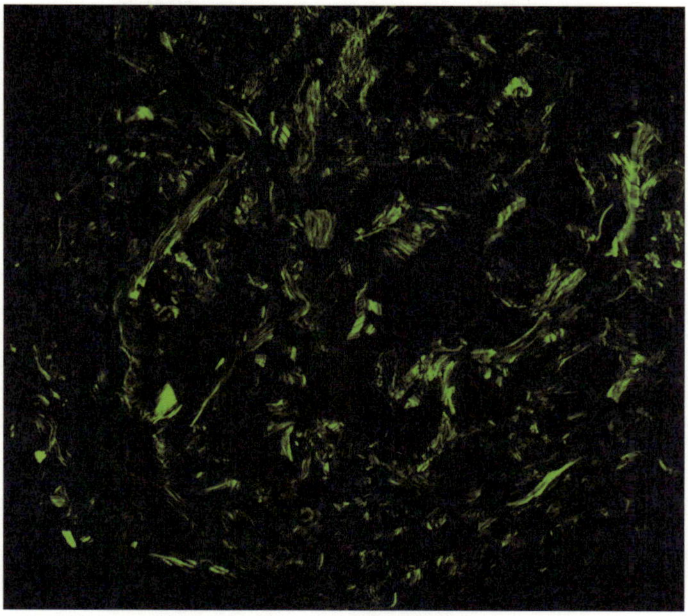

Figure 8.
Laser scanning confocal microscopic study using second-harmonic generation technique reveals the structure of collagen fibrils in acellular dermal matrix after decellularization and X-ray radiation 35 kG (Bar 1/4 50 mm).

4. Conclusion

To date, there is no causative treatment of EB, despite multiple ongoing studies involving gene therapy and bone marrow transplantation. The standard of EB management still involves symptomatic conservative treatment. There is immense hope in therapies with the use of stem cells of various origins (bone marrow, umbilical cord, etc.). Advanced applications of various types of cells (embryonic, prenatal, and adult stem cells, endothelial cells, and melanocytes) and the rapid development of biomedical engineering, which contributes to refining biocompatible materials, such as collagen, hyaluronic acid, elastin, polylactic acid (PLA), poly lactic-co-glycolic acid (PLGA), and polyethylene glycol (PEG), bring hope of effective treatment for chronic wounds of various origin. The most recent developments allow for the manufacture of progressively better skin substitutes, which in the future may exhibit the fundamental characteristics of natural human skin (including sweat glands and hair follicles), more homogeneous pigmentation, and allow for the healing of scars [65]. Thus, further studies and efforts are crucial for creating skin substitutes truly mimicking natural skin. Despite the enormous progress in the treatment of EB, the current treatments are clearly not a definitive cure for this debilitating disease, and the risk associated with some of these procedures must be weighed against their potential benefits. Effective treatment of this, currently incurable, group of diseases requires advanced and innovative strategies with an improved safety profile, such as the ones that are currently being developed [66–77].

The BiOOPA dressing is easily available, safe, and relatively inexpensive, all of which make it a promising therapy for EB-associated wounds. Preliminary results of the BIOOPA study indicate the dressing to be safe and effective to improve the quality of life in study subjects. Currently BIOOPA is evaluated as part of a phase

I/II clinical study during the second year of observation. Our preliminary results of clinical trial strongly suggest, that our innovative dressing is a promising strategy and a tool for clinicians in the search for new opportunities of treatment for this rare condition.

Acknowledgements

This is unpublished Original Article.The study has been approved by an ethics committee (KB/ 2019 14/01/2019; KB/177/2015). Supported by The National Center for Research and Development in terms of the project “Prevention Practices and Treatment of Civilizations Diseases-STRATEGMED” (grant no. STRATERMED2/ 269807/14/NCBR/2015).

EudraCT Number: 2018-003890-91.

Protocol number BIOOPA DBL.474.317.2020.

Author details

Magdalena Nita[1], Jacek Pliszczyński[1], Andrzej Eljaszewicz[2], Marcin Moniuszko[2,3], Tomasz Ołdak[4], Katarzyna Woźniak[5], Sławomir Majewski[6], Cezary Kowalewski[5], Artur Kamiński[7], Dariusz Śladowski[7], Zbigniew Zimek[8], Maciej Kosieradzki[1] and Piotr Fiedor[1*]

1 Department of General and Transplantation Surgery at Medical University of Warsaw, Infant Jesus Clinical Hospital, Warsaw, Poland

2 Department of Regenerative Medicine and Immune Regulation at Medical University of Białystok, Białystok, Poland

3 Department of Allergology and Internal Medicine at Medical University of Białystok, Białystok, Poland

4 PBKM, Polish Stem Cells Bank, Warsaw, Poland

5 Department of Dermatology and Immunodermatology at Medical University of Warsaw, Warsaw, Poland

6 Department of Dermatology and Venereology at Medical University of Warsaw, Warsaw, Poland

7 Department of Transplantology and Central Tissue Bank at Medical University of Warsaw, Warsaw, Poland

8 Institute of Nuclear Chemistry and Technology, Warsaw, Poland

*Address all correspondence to: piotrfiedor@wp.pl

References

[1] Epidermolysis bullosa – pęcherzowe oddzielanie się naskórka. Etiopatogeneza, dziedziczenie, diagnostyka, leczenie.Katarzyna Wertheim-Tysarowska, Cezary Kowalewski, Katarzyna Woźniak, Jerzy Bal, Wyd. Continuo;

[2] Genetyczne uwarunkowanie choroby skóry-przegląd wybranych genodermatoz, Medycyna Wieku Rozwojowego, 2012, XVI, 3, © IMiD, Wydawnictwo Aluna.

[3] Tantcheva-Poór I, Oji V, Has C (2016) A multistep approach to the diagnosis of rare genodermatoses. J Dtsch Dermatol Ges 14: 969-986 2. www.genodermatoses-network.org

[4] Schaffer JV (2016) Practice and Educational Gaps in Genodermatoses. Dermatol Clin 34: 303-310

[5] Smith FJD, McLean WHI (2011) Genodermatoses: Inherited Deisease of the Skin, W: Murphy MJ (red) Molecular Diagnostics in Dermatology and Dermatopathology, Estados Unidos : Humana Press, str 379- 410

[6] Jabłońska S, Majewski S (2006) Budowa i czynności skóry W: Jabłońska S, Majewski S (red) Choroby skóry i choroby przenoszone drogą płciową PZWL, str 15-28

[7] Tsuruta D, Hashimoto T, Hamill KJ, Jones JC (2011) Hemidesmosomes and focal contact proteins: functions and cross-talk in keratinocytes, bullous diseases and wound healing. J Dermatol Sci 62: 1-7

[8] Green KJ, Simpson CL (2007) Desmosomes: new perspectives on a classic. J Invest Dermatol 127: 2499-2515

[9] Coulombe PA, Kerns ML, Fuchs E (2009) Epidermolysis bullosa simplex: a paradigm for disorders of tissue fragility. J Clin Invest 119: 1784-1793

[10] Fine JD, General cutaneous manifestations (2009), W: Fine JD, Hintner H (red) Life with Epidermolysis Bullosa, SpringerWienNewYork, str 99-106

[11] Fine JD, Johnson LB, Weiner M, Li KP, Suchindran C (2009) Epidermolysis bullosa and the risk of life-threatening cancers: the National EB Registry experience, 1986-2006 J Am Acad Dermatol 60: 203-211

[12] Fine JD, Other internal complications (2009), W: Fine JD, Hintner H (red) Life with Epidermolysis Bullosa, SpringerWienNewYork; str 185-196

[13] Fine JD, Bruckner-Tuderman L, Eady RA, Bauer EA, Bauer JW, Has C, Heagerty A, Hintner H, Hovnanian A, Jonkman MF, Leigh I, Marinkovich MP, Martinez AE, McGrath JA, Mellerio JE, Moss C, Murrell DF, Shimizu H, Uitto J, Woodley D, Zambruno G (2014). Inherited epidermolysis bullosa: updated recommendations on diagnosis and classification. J Am Acad Dermatol 70: 1103-1126 14.

[14] Has C (2018) Advances in understanding the molecular basis of skin fragility. F1000Res 7: 279

[15] Wertheim-Tysarowska K, Ołdak M, Giza A, Kutkowska-Kaźmierczak A, Sota J, Przybylska D, Woźniak K, Śniegórska D, Niepokój K, Sobczyńska-Tomaszewska A, Rygiel AM, Płoski R, Bal J, Kowalewski C (2016) Novel sporadic and recurrent mutations in KRT5 and KRT14 genes in Polish epidermolysis bullosa simplex patients: further insights into epidemiology and genotype-phenotype correlation. J Appl Genet 57: 175-81

[16] Bardhan, A., Bruckner-Tuderman, L., Chapple, I. L. C., Fine, J.-D., Harper, N., Has, C., ... Heagerty, A. H. (2020).

Epidermolysis bullosa. Nature Reviews Disease Primers, 6(1). doi:10.1038/s41572-020-0210-0

[17] Blount AL, Foster S, Rapp DA, et al. The use of bioelectric dressings in skin graft harvest sites: a prospective case series. J Burn Care Res. 2012;33:354–357.

[18] Goertz O, Abels C, Knie U, et al. Clinical safety and efficacy of a novel thermoreversible polyhexanide-preserved wound covering gel. Eur Surg Res. 2010;44:96–101.

[19] Hasatsri S, Angspatt A, Aramwit P. Randomized clinical trial of the innovative bilayered wound dressing made of silk and gela- tin: safety and efficacy tests using a split-thickness skin graft mod- el. Evid Based Complement Alternat Med. 2015;2015:206871.

[20] Metelmann HR, Brandner J, Schumann H, et al. Accelerating the aesthetic benefit of wound healing by triterpene. J Craniomaxillofac Surg. 2012;40:e150–e154.

[21] Potocká D, Kevická D, Koller J. Clinical trial of the temporary biosynthetic dermal skin substitute based on a collagen and hy- aluronic acid named Coladerm H/HM, first part. Acta Chir Plast. 2012;54:31–38.

[22] Baser NT, Yuksel A, Unzile B, et al. High-valve vapor-permeable film dressing versus fine mesh gauze dressing on skin graft donor areas in diabetic patients: a prospective randomized controlled trial. European J Plast Surg. 2008;31:219–228.

[23] Siritientong T, Angspatt A, Ratanavaraporn J, et al. Clinical potential of a silk sericin-releasing bioactive wound dressing for the treatment of split-thickness skin graft donor sites. Pharm Res. 2014;31: 104–116.

[24] Junker JP, Kamel RA, Caterson EJ, et al. Clinical impact upon wound healing and inflammation in moist, wet, and dry environ- ments Adv Wound Care (New Rochelle). 2013;2:348–356.

[25] Rakel BA, Bermel MA, Abbott LI, et al. Split-thickness skin graft donor site care: a quantitative synthesis of the research. Appl Nurs Res. 1998;11:174–182.

[26] Wiechula R. The use of moist wound-healing dressings in the management of split-thickness skin graft donor sites: a systematic review. Int J Nurs Pract. 2003;9:S9–17.

[27] Moher D, Shamseer L, Clarke M, et al.; PRISMA-P Group. Preferred reporting items for systematic review and meta-analysis protocols (PRISMA-P) 2015 statement. Syst Rev. 2015;4:1.

[28] Fine JD. Musculoskeletal deformities. In: Fine JD, Hintner H: Life with epidermolysis bullosa (EB): Etiology, diagnosis, multidisciplinary patient care, and therapy. Wien, NewYork: Springer, 2009: 178–84.

[29] Rees TD, Swinyard A. Rehabilitative digital surgery in epidermolysis bullosa. Plast Reconstr Surg 1967;40(2):169–74.

[30] Vozdivzhensky SI, Albanova VI. Surgical treatment of contracture and syndactyly of children with epidermolysis bullosa. Br J Plast Surg 1993; 46:314–6.

[31] Ciccarelli AO, Rothaus KO, Carter DM, et al. Plastic and reconstructive surgery in epidermolysis bullosa: clinical experience with 110 procedures in 25 patients. Ann Plast Surg 1995;35:254–61.

[32] Siprashvili, Z., Nguyen, N. T., Gorell, E. S., Loutit, K., Khuu, P., Furukawa, L. K., ... Marinkovich, M. P. (2016). Safety and Wound Outcomes Following Genetically Corrected Autologous Epidermal Grafts in Patients With Recessive Dystrophic

Epidermolysis Bullosa. JAMA, 316(17), 1808. doi:10.1001/jama.2016.15588

[33] Kühl, T., Mezger, M., Hausser, I., Guey, L. T., Handgretinger, R., Bruckner-Tuderman, L., & Nyström, A. (2016). Collagen VII Half-Life at the Dermal-Epidermal Junction Zone: Implications for Mechanisms and Therapy of Genodermatoses. Journal of Investigative Dermatology, 136(6), 1116–1123. doi:10.1016/j.jid.2016.02.002

[34] Nekanti, U., Rao, V. B., Bahirvani, A. G., Jan, M., Totey, S., & Ta, M. (2010). Long-Term Expansion and Pluripotent Marker Array Analysis of Wharton's Jelly-Derived Mesenchymal Stem Cells. Stem Cells and Development, 19(1), 117–130. doi: 10.1089/scd.2009.0177

[35] Karahuseyinoglu, S., Cinar, O., Kilic, E., Kara, F., Akay, G. G., Demiralp, D. Ö., ... Can, A. (2007). Biology of Stem Cells in Human Umbilical Cord Stroma: In Situ and In Vitro Surveys. Stem Cells, 25(2), 319–331. doi:10.1634/stemcells.2006-0286

[36] Tipnis, S., Viswanathan, C., & Majumdar, A. S. (2010). Immunosuppressive properties of human umbilical cord-derived mesenchymal stem cells: role of B7-H1 and IDO. Immunology and Cell Biology, 88(8), 795–806. doi:10.1038/icb.2010.47

[37] Shen, Y., Zhu, Y.-M., Fan, X., Shi, J.-Y., Wang, Q.-R., Yan, X.-J., ... Chen, S.-J. (2011). Gene mutation patterns and their prognostic impact in a cohort of 1185 patients with acute myeloid leukemia. Blood, 118(20), 5593–5603. doi:10.1182/blood-2011-03-343988

[38] Choi, S.-E., & Kemper, J. K. (2013). Regulation of SIRT1 by MicroRNAs. Molecules and Cells, 36(5), 385–392. doi: 10.1007/s10059-013-0297-1.

[39] Nekanti, U., Mohanty, L., Venugopal, P., Balasubramanian, S., Totey, S., & Ta, M. (2010). Optimization and scale-up of Wharton's jelly-derived mesenchymal stem cells for clinical applications. Stem Cell Research, 5(3), 244–254. doi:10.1016/j.scr.2010.08.005

[40] Koster MI (2009) Making an epidermis. Ann N Y Acad Sci 1170: 7-10

[41] Chen, H., Wang, W., Xie, H., Xu, X., Wu, J., Jiang, Z., ... Zheng, S. (2009). A pathogenic role of IL- 17 at the early stage of corneal allograft rejection. Transplant Immunology, 21 (3), 155–161. doi:10.1016/j.trim.2009.03.006

[42] Gough MJ, Page RE. Surgical correction of the hand in epidermolysis bullosa dystrophica. Hand 1979; 11(1): 55–8.

[43] Eastwood DS. Autografting in the treatment of squa- mous cell carcinoma in epidermolysis bullosa dys- trophica. Plast Reconstr Surg 1972;49(1):93–5.

[44] Eisenberg M, Llewelyn D. Surgical management of hands in children with recessive dystrophic epider- molysis bullosa: use of allogeneic composite cultured skin grafts. Br J Plast Surg 19 Damanhuri M, Boyle J, Enoch S (2011) Advances in tissue-engineered skin substitutes. Wounds Int 2 (1):27–34

[45] Nicholas MN, Yeung J (2017a) Current status and future of skin substitutes for chronic wound healing. J Cutan Med Surg 21(1):23–30

[46] Nicholas MN, Jeschke MG, Amini-Nik S (2016a) Cellularized bilayer pullulan-gelatin hydrogel for skin regeneration. Tissue Eng A 22(9–10): 754–764

[47] Sheikholeslam M, Wright ME, Jeschke MG, Amini-Nik S (2017) Biomaterials for Skin Substitutes. AdvHealthcare Mater

[48] MacNeil S (2007) Progress and opportunities for tissue- engineered skin. Nature 445(7130):874

[49] Böttcher-Haberzeth S, Klar AS, Biedermann T, Schiestl C, Meuli-Simmen C, Reichmann E, Meuli M (2013) "Trooping the color": restoring the original donor skin color by addition of melanocytes to bioengineered skin analogs. Pediatr Surg Int29(3):239–247

[50] Biedermann T, Boettcher-Haberzeth S, Reichmann E (2013) Tissue engineering of skin for wound coverage. Eur J PediatrSurg 23(5):375–382

[51] Lovett M, Lee K, Edwards A, Kaplan DL (2009) Vascularization strategies for tissue engineering. Tissue Eng B Rev 15 (3):353–370

[52] Catalano E, Cochis A, Varoni E, Rimondini L, Azzimonti B (2013) Tissue-engineered skin substitutes: an over- view. J ArtifOrgans 16(4):397–403 98;51:608–13

[53] Damanhuri M, Boyle J, Enoch S (2011) Advances in tissue-engineered skin substitutes. Wounds Int 2 (1):27–34

[54] Supp, D. M. & Boyce, S. T. 2005 Engineered skin substitutes: practices and potentials. Clin. Dermatol. 23, 403–412. (doi:10.1016/j.clindermatol.2004.07.023)

[55] Halim AS, Khoo TL, Mohd Yussof SJ (2010a) Biologic and synthetic skin substitutes: An overview. Indian J Plast Surg 43(Suppl):S23–S28

[56] Halim AS, Khoo TL, Yussof SJM (2010b) Biologic and synthetic skin substitutes: an overview. Indian J Plastic Surg 43(Suppl):S23

[57] Lepow, B. D., Downey, M., Yurgelon, J., Klassen, L., & Armstrong, D. G. (2011). Bioengineered tissues in wound healing: a progress report. Expert Review of Dermatology, 6(3), 255–262. doi:10.1586/edm.11.27

[58] Varkey M, Ding J, Tredget EE (2015a) Advances in skin substitutes-potential of tissue engineered skin for facilitating antifibrotic healing. J Funct Biomater 6 (3):547–563

[59] Varkey, M., Ding, J., & Tredget, E. (2015). Advances in Skin Substitutes—Potential of Tissue Engineered Skin for Facilitating Anti-Fibrotic Healing. Journal of Functional Biomaterials, 6(3), 547–563. doi:10.3390/jfb6030547

[60] Jutkiewicz, J., Noszczyk, B. H., & Wrobel, M. (2010). The use of Biobrane for hand surgery in Epidermolysis bullosa. Journal of Plastic, Reconstructive & Aesthetic Surgery, 63 (8), 1305–1311. doi:10.1016/j.bjps.2009.06.038

[61] Fivenson DP, Scherschun L, Cohen LV. Apligraf in the treatment of severe mitten deformity associated with recessive dystrophic epidermolysis bullosa. Plast Reconstr Surg 2003;112 (2):584–8.

[62] Falabella, A. F., Valencia, I. C., Eaglstein, W. H., & Schachner, L. A. (2000). Tissue-Engineered Skin (Apligraf) in the Healing of Patients With Epidermolysis Bullosa Wounds. Archives of Dermatology, 136(10). doi: 10.1001/archderm.136.10.1225

[63] Nita, M., Pliszczyński, J., Kowalewski, C., Woźniak, K., Eljaszewicz, A., Moniuszko, M., Fiedor, P. (2020). New Treatment of Wound Healing With Allogenic Acellular Human Skin Graft: Preclinical Assessment and In Vitro Study. Transplantation Proceedings. doi: 10.1016/j.transproceed.2020.02.115

[64] Pliszczyński, J., Nita, M., Kowalewski, C., Woźniak, K., Eljaszewicz, A., Moniuszko, M., Fiedor, P. (2020). Transplantation of a New

Biological Product in Rare Diseases, Such as Epidermolysis Bullosa: Response and Clinical Outcome. Transplantation Proceedings. doi:10.1016/j.transproceed.2020.02.119

[65] MacNeil S (2008) Biomaterials for tissue engineering of skin. Mater Today 11(5):26–35

[66] Conget P, Rodriguez F, Kramer S, et al. Replenishment of type VII collagen and re-epithelialization of chronically ulcerated skin after intradermal administration of allogeneic mesenchymal stromal cells in two patients with recessive dystrophic epidermolysis bullosa. Cytotherapy 2010;12:429–31.

[67] Abe R, Donnelly SC, Peng T, Bucala R, Metz CN. Peripheral blood fibrocytes: differentiation pathway and migration to wound sites. J Immunol 2001;166: 7556–62.

[68] Ito M, Liu Y, Yang Z, et al. Stem cells in the hair follicle bulge contribute to wound repair but not to homeostasis of the epidermis. Nat Med 2005;11: 1351–4.

[69] Leoni G, Neumann PA, Sumagin R, Denning TL, Nusrat A. Wound repair: role of immune-epithelial interactions. Mucosal Immunol 2015;8: 959–68.

[70] Badiavas EV, Abedi M, Butmarc J, Falanga V, Quesenberry P. Participation of bone marrow derived cells in cutaneous wound healing. J Cell Physiol 2003;196:245–50.

[71] Sasaki M, Abe R, Fujita Y, Ando S, Inokuma D, Shimizu H. Mesenchymal stem cells are recruited into wounded skin and contribute to wound repair by transdifferentiation into multiple skin cell type. J Immunol 2008;180:2581–7.

[72] Inokuma D, Abe R, Fujita Y, et al. CTACK/CCL27 accelerates skin regeneration via accumulation of bone marrow-derivedkeratinocytes. Stem Cells 2006;24:2810–6.

[73] Sebastiano V, Zhen HH, Haddad B, Bashkirova E, Melo SP, Wang P, Leung TL, Siprashvili Z, Tichy A, Li J, Ameen M, Hawkins J, Lee S, Li L, Schwertschkow A, Bauer G, Lisowski L, Kay MA, Kim SK, Lane AT, Wernig M, Oro AE; Human COL7A1-corrected induced pluripotent stem cells for the treatment of recessive dystrophic epidermolysis bullosa. Sci Transl Med. 2014 Nov 26; 6(264):264ra163.

[74] Takahashi K, Tanabe K, Ohnuki M, Narita M, Ichisaka T, Tomoda K, Yamanaka S, Induction of pluripotent stem cells from adult human fibroblasts by defined factors Cell. 2007 Nov 30; 131(5):861-72

[75] S Spiliopoulos, N Davans,Induced pluripotent stem cells for the treatment of recessive dystrophic epidermolysis bullosa. Ann Transl Med. 2015 Dec;3 (22):349. doi: 10.3978/j.issn.2305-5839.2015.09.42.

[76] Horwitz EM, Prockop DJ, Gordon PL, Koo WW, Fitzpatrick LA, Neel MD, McCarville ME, Orchard PJ, Pyeritz RE, Brenner MK. Clinical responses to bone marrow transplantation in children with severe osteogenesis imperfecta. Blood. 2001 Mar 1;97(5):1227-31.

[77] Dominici M, Marino R, Rasini V, Spano C, Paolucci P, Conte P, Hofmann TJ,Horwitz EM. Donor cell-derived osteopoiesis originates from a self-renewing stem cell with a limited regenerative contribution after transplantation. Blood. 2008 Apr 15;111 (8):4386-91. doi: 10.1182/blood-2007-10-115725. Epub 2008 Jan 8.